To read before

becoming a

Nursing assistant

in Dermatology

MARTIN STERLING

Table of contents

"*The skin is our first contact with the world, and dermatology is its map, tracing the paths of health, beauty and identity.*

Chapter 1:
INTRODUCTION TO DERMATOLOGY

Definition and brief history dermatology

Dermatology is the branch of medicine devoted to the study, diagnosis, prevention and treatment of diseases of the skin, mucous membranes, nails and hair. It also covers aesthetic, cosmetic and venereal (sexually transmitted) disorders. The dermatologist is the specialist doctor who practises this discipline, and his field of action is vast, ranging from benign conditions such as acne or eczema to skin cancers.

<u>A brief history of dermatology</u>

Antiquity
The first references to skin diseases date back to ancient times. Egyptian papyri dating from 1500 BC already describe symptoms similar to those of skin diseases known today. Hippocrates, the father of modern medicine, listed numerous skin conditions in his writings.

The Middle Ages
In the Middle Ages, leprosy was one of the most feared skin diseases, leading to patients being isolated in leper colonies. Doctors of the time used plant- and mineral-based concoctions to treat various skin conditions, although their effectiveness was largely empirical.

Renaissance
It was during the Renaissance that medicine began to adopt a more scientific approach. Artists such as Leonardo

da Vinci studied human anatomy, which indirectly contributed to a better understanding of the skin.

18th and 19th centuries
Dermatology began to emerge as a distinct speciality in the 18th century. With the advent of microscopy, researchers were able to study the skin at a cellular level, which led to a better understanding of skin diseases. In the 19th century, the classification of dermatological diseases became more structured, and the first dermatological clinics were established.

20th century to the present day
The 20th century saw major innovations in the field of dermatology. The discovery of antibiotics revolutionised the treatment of many infectious skin conditions. Aesthetic dermatology, with procedures such as plastic surgery, botox and dermal fillers, also became popular. Today, with the advent of molecular biology and genetics, dermatology continues to evolve, allowing more targeted and effective treatments for a variety of skin conditions.

Dermatology is a rich medical speciality that has evolved over the centuries. From the empirical observation of symptoms to the molecular understanding of diseases, this discipline continues to provide solutions to the challenges posed by skin, hair and nail disorders.

The importance of dermatology in the medical world

As a medical discipline, dermatology plays an essential role in the overall care of patients. Its importance goes far beyond the simple treatment of skin disorders. Here are a few points that underline the vital importance of dermatology in the medical world:

1. The omnipresence of skin
The skin is the largest organ in the human body, serving as the first line of defence against pathogens and other environmental threats. It also plays a crucial role in regulating body temperature, protecting against UV rays, and sensory perception. Healthy skin is therefore vital to our overall well-being.

2. Overall health indicator
Many internal diseases manifest themselves through skin symptoms. Conditions such as lupus, diabetes and thyroid disease can have dermatological manifestations. As a result, the dermatologist is often the first doctor to diagnose these systemic diseases.

3. Prevention and detection of skin cancers
Skin cancer is one of the most common cancers in many countries. Thanks to dermatology, skin cancers such as melanoma can be detected at an early stage, increasing the chances of recovery. Prevention through education about sun protection is also a fundamental aspect of the discipline.

4. Quality of life
Skin conditions, even benign ones such as eczema or psoriasis, can have a significant impact on patients' quality of life. Pain, itching and cosmetic concerns can lead to sleep disturbance, stress and anxiety. Dermatology offers solutions to improve patients' well-being.

5. Innovation and research
Dermatology is at the forefront of many medical innovations, from topical treatments to laser surgery and gene therapies. Dermatology research is dynamic, with a constant quest for better solutions to treat skin conditions.

6. Interface between medicine and cosmetology
Dermatology is unique in that it straddles the fields of pure medicine and cosmetology. Dermatologists are often involved in aesthetic treatments, helping patients to feel better about themselves, both literally and figuratively.

Dermatology is therefore a key medical discipline, playing a central role in the prevention, diagnosis and treatment of a multitude of conditions. It represents an interface between overall health, physical and psychological well-being, and aesthetics, underlining its multidimensional importance in the medical world.

Common pathologies in dermatology

Dermatology treats a wide range of skin conditions. These conditions vary according to their severity, symptoms and causes. Here is a list of the most common skin conditions treated in dermatology:

1. Acne
   - **Description**: Skin condition manifested by pimples, blackheads, cysts and nodules.
   - **Causes**: Hormones, bacteria, excessive sebum secretion, genetic factors.

2. Eczema (atopic dermatitis)
   - **Description**: Dry, red, itchy skin that can lead to lesions following scratching.
   - **Causes**: Allergic reactions, genetic, environmental and immune factors.

3. Psoriasis
   - **Description:** Thick, red, scaly patches on the skin.

- **Causes**: Autoimmune disease, can be triggered by factors such as stress, certain infections or medication.

4. Vitiligo
- **Description**: Loss of skin pigmentation forming discoloured areas.
- **Causes**: Autoimmune disease in which the immune system attacks the pigment cells.

5. Rosacea
- **Description**: Redness, small visible vessels and, sometimes, the appearance of pimples on the face.
- **Causes**: Genetic, vascular and inflammatory factors.

6. Herpes
- **Description**: Small, painful vesicles, often grouped in clusters, usually on or around the lips or genitals.
- **Causes**: Viruses (HSV-1 for the labial type and HSV-2 for the genital type).

7. Skin mycoses
- **Description**: Skin infections caused by fungi.
- **Causes**: Various types of fungi, such as dermatophytes or candida.

8. Warts
- **Description**: Rough, generally painless growths on the skin or mucous membranes.
- **Causes**: Human papillomavirus (HPV).

9. Contact dermatitis
- **Description**: Redness, itching and sometimes blisters on the skin.
- **Causes**: Allergic or irritant reaction to an external substance (allergens or irritants).

10. Skin cancer
- Common types :
- **Basal cell carcinoma: the** most common form, but generally non-metastatic.
- **Squamous cell carcinoma:** potentially more aggressive than basal cell carcinoma.
- **Melanoma**: pigmented skin cancer, potentially very aggressive.

11. Urticaria
- **Description**: Raised red patches accompanied by itching.
- **Causes**: Allergic reactions, infections, medication, stress or other triggers.

12. Angiomas
- **Description**: Red or purple patches due to dilated blood vessels.
- **Types** : Stellate angiomas, haemangiomas.

These conditions represent a fraction of the diseases treated in dermatology. Each presents its own diagnostic and treatment challenges. Thanks to ongoing research and innovation in dermatology, many therapeutic options are available to manage and treat these conditions.

Chapter 2:
THE DERMATOLOGY ORDERLY: A KEY ROLE

General presentation
the nursing auxiliary profession

Healthcare assistants occupy a central position in the healthcare system. They generally work closely with nursing and medical staff to provide basic patient care. Here is an overview of the nursing auxiliary profession, its responsibilities, training and role in the healthcare system.

1. Role and responsibilities
Healthcare assistants are mainly responsible for :

- **Basic care**: This involves helping patients with their daily activities, including washing, dressing, moving around, eating, etc.
- **Monitoring**: This involves monitoring the patient's general condition, taking vital signs such as temperature, pulse and blood pressure, and passing on the relevant information to nursing or medical staff.
- **Hygiene and comfort**: Ensures that the patient's environment is clean and safe. They change sheets, clean rooms and disinfect if necessary.
- **Communication**: The nursing auxiliary is often the first point of contact for the patient. They listen, reassure, inform and play a crucial role in the patient's psychological well-being.

2. Training and skills
Training to become a nursing auxiliary is generally shorter than that for nurses. It includes :

- **Theoretical training**: This covers the fundamentals of care, anatomy, physiology, etc.
- **Clinical placements**: Clinical placements enable trainee nursing assistants to gain practical experience in a range of care services and facilities.
- **Essential qualities**: empathy, patience, physical stamina, listening skills, ability to work in a team and adaptability.

3. Working environment

Healthcare assistants can work in a variety of environments, such as :

- **Hospitals**: In various departments such as surgery, paediatrics, geriatrics, dermatology, etc.
- **Establishments for the elderly**: retirement homes, EHPAD (Etablissements d'Hébergement pour Personnes Âgées Dépendantes), etc.
- **Homecare services**: Providing care to patients in their own homes.
- **Rehabilitation or re-education centres**: For patients requiring physical or functional re-education.

4. Outlook and developments

The nursing auxiliary profession is often seen as a first step into the medical field. Many then choose to continue their training to become nurses, specialist nurses or even health managers. There are plenty of opportunities for advancement, provided you keep up to date with training and adapt to the changing demands of the profession.

The profession of care assistant is essential to guaranteeing quality patient care. It requires dedication, skill and compassion. The care assistant is the pillar on which the comfort and well-being of the patient rests during his or her stay in a care facility.

Special features the role of dermatology

Dermatology, which focuses on the care and treatment of the skin, presents a number of challenges and specificities that require particular skills on the part of healthcare assistants. Working on the front line, the dermatology orderly plays a vital role in the overall care of patients with skin conditions. Let's take a closer look at the specifics of this role.

1. Understanding skin pathologies
   - **Awareness**: Knowledge of common skin conditions such as eczema, psoriasis, acne, fungal infections, skin cancers, etc.
   - **Symptom recognition**: Ability to identify signs of worsening or improvement in a dermatological condition, so as to quickly inform the medical team.

2. Specific care and techniques
   - **Local treatment**: Application of creams, ointments, lotions, special bandages, etc. as prescribed and under the direction of the nurse or dermatologist.
   - **Dressing management**: Technique for applying, removing and caring for specific dressings for skin ulcers, biopsies, minor surgery, etc.

3. Patient education and advice
   - **Hygiene advice**: Inform patients on how to clean and care for their skin, especially when it is affected by a dermatological condition.
   - **Application of treatments**: Advise and educate the patient on how to correctly apply topical treatments.

4. Sensitivity and psychological support
  * **Empathy**: Many skin conditions can have a significant impact on self-esteem. The carer must therefore be a good listener, reassuring and non-judgemental.
  * **Support**: Providing emotional support to patients, especially those who may be stigmatised or have a difficult time coping with their skin condition.

5. Hygiene and prevention measures
  * **Infection prevention**: Ensure that wounds and skin conditions are properly cleaned and protected to avoid any risk of secondary infection.
  * **Sun protection**: Educate patients about the importance of sun protection, particularly when using photosensitising treatments or if they have a history of skin cancer.

6. Close collaboration with the medical team
  * **Communication**: Passing on all relevant information about the patient's condition to the medical team, particularly nurses and dermatologists.
  * **Participation in consultations**: Assisting with dermatology consultations to help implement procedures or manage patients.

The role of the dermatology orderly is both demanding and rewarding. It requires a combination of technical skills, in-depth knowledge of skin conditions, and a great deal of empathy and psychological support. This specialisation enables the nursing assistant to have a direct and positive impact on patients' quality of life.

The qualities required to excel in this field

Excelling as a care assistant in the field of dermatology requires a set of specific skills and personal qualities. These qualities go beyond technical and clinical training. They encompass character traits and attitudes that guarantee optimal care for patients with skin disorders.

1. Empathy and compassion
   - **Understanding emotions**: Many dermatological conditions can affect a patient's self-esteem. Being able to understand and feel what patients are going through is crucial.
   - **Reassuring attitude**: Bringing comfort and reassurance to patients, especially those who are anxious or worried about their condition.

2. Sense of detail
   - **Careful observation**: Being able to spot subtle changes in the skin or in the condition of a lesion can make a big difference to patient care.
   - **Precise application**: Ensuring that treatments are applied correctly and according to instructions.

3. Patience
   - **Managing repetition**: Some care and treatment needs to be administered regularly and can be repetitive.
   - **Ongoing support**: Be patient with those who are frustrated or discouraged by the pace of their recovery.

4. Excellent communication skills
   - **Active listening**: knowing how to listen to patients' concerns and questions, without interrupting them or minimising their feelings.

- **Passing on information**: Being able to clearly explain procedures, care and advice to patients.

5. Integrity and professionalism
  - **Confidentiality**: Respecting patients' privacy and dignity by keeping their medical information confidential.
  - **Commitment**: To be dedicated to providing quality care and acting in the best interests of the patient.

6. Physical and mental endurance
  - **Resilience**: Being able to manage stress and pressure in an often busy medical environment.
  - **Physical strength**: In some cases, helping patients to move or move around may require a certain amount of strength and stamina.

7. Adaptability
  - **Continuous learning**: Dermatology, like all medical fields, is constantly evolving. Nurses must be ready to learn and adapt to new techniques and knowledge.
  - **Handling unexpected situations**: Knowing how to react calmly and effectively in an emergency or unexpected situation.

8. Teamwork
  - **Collaboration**: Working effectively with dermatologists, nurses and the rest of the medical team to ensure comprehensive patient care.
  - **Positive attitude**: Contributing to a harmonious and productive working atmosphere.

To excel as a dermatology orderly, you need not only clinical skills, but also a range of human qualities. The combination of these qualities ensures that patients are cared for comprehensively and humanely, promoting their well-being and recovery.

Chapter 3:
TECHNIQUES AND FUNDAMENTAL PROCEDURES

The basics of disinfection and asepsis in dermatology

In dermatology, as in all medical fields, maintaining a sterile environment is essential to prevent the spread of infections. This is all the more crucial when dealing with the skin, which is the body's first line of defence against pathogens. Here's an overview of the basics of disinfection and asepsis specific to dermatology.

1. Key definitions
   - **Disinfection**: Process that eliminates most or all pathogenic micro-organisms from an object or surface, with the exception of bacterial spores.
   - **Asepsis**: Prevention of the entry of pathogenic micro-organisms into a sterile environment or site, such as a wound or incision.

2. Importance of asepsis in dermatology
   - **Damaged skin**: Damaged or altered skin is more vulnerable to infection. It is therefore crucial to ensure that all tools and surfaces that come into contact with the skin are sterile.
   - **Invasive procedures**: Biopsies, excisions and other dermatological procedures can introduce pathogens into the body if strict standards of asepsis are not observed.

3. Disinfection techniques
- **Cleaning**: Mechanical removal of dirt and most micro-organisms. This is the first stage before disinfection.
- **Antiseptics**: Substances applied to the skin to reduce the presence of micro-organisms. Examples: alcohol, povidone-iodine.
- **Disinfectants** : Substances used to disinfect surfaces and medical equipment. They are not intended for use on the skin. Examples: bleach, hydrogen peroxide.

4. Asepsis during dermatological procedures
- **Preparing the skin**: The area to be treated must be thoroughly cleaned and disinfected before any procedure.
- **Sterile gloves**: These must be worn during invasive procedures to avoid contamination.
- **Sterilisation of instruments** : Instruments that penetrate the skin (needles, scalpels, etc.) must be sterilised, generally by autoclaving.
- **No-touch techniques**: Where possible, use techniques that minimise or eliminate direct contact with non-sterile areas.

5. Preventing cross-contamination
- **Single use**: Use single-use materials (needles, blades, etc.) whenever possible.
- **Hand washing**: This is the most basic and effective measure for preventing the spread of infections.
- **Appropriate disposal** : Sharps and any contaminated material must be disposed of safely, following established protocols.

6. Patient education
- **Post-procedure care**: Informing patients on how to take care of their skin after a procedure to avoid infections.

- **Recognising the signs of infection**: Educate patients about the signs of infection, such as redness, swelling, warmth, pus or increased pain, and tell them when to seek medical attention.

Compliance with asepsis and disinfection protocols in dermatology is essential to guarantee patient safety and avoid complications. Whether during a simple consultation or a surgical operation, these principles remain fundamental and must be rigorously applied.

Preparing the patient for the examination

The dermatological examination is a crucial step in diagnosing and treating skin disorders. Proper preparation of the patient is necessary to obtain optimal results and to ensure patient comfort during the examination. Here is an overview of the essential steps in preparing a patient for a dermatological examination.

1. Initial communication
   - **Explanation of the process**: Inform the patient how the examination will be carried out, how long it will take and which areas will be examined.
   - **Reassuring the patient**: Some patients may be anxious or embarrassed. It is important to reassure them and establish a relationship of trust.

2. Medical history
   - **General information**: Collect essential data, such as age, sex, medical and surgical history.
   - **Dermatological history**: Investigate previous skin conditions, treatments undergone and their results.

3. Physical preparation
- **Clothing**: Ask the patient to remove all clothing except underwear and put on a medical gown.
- **Jewellery and accessories**: Ask the patient to remove all jewellery, watches, piercings and other objects that could interfere with the examination.
- **Cleaning the skin**: If necessary, provide cleansing wipes so that the patient can remove any residue of cream, make-up or lotion from the area to be examined.

4. Setting up the environment
- **Lighting**: Ensure appropriate lighting for close observation of the skin.
- **Privacy**: Use screens or curtains to ensure the patient's privacy during the examination.
- **Room temperature**: Maintain a comfortable temperature to prevent the patient becoming too cold when undressed.

5. Instrument preparation
- **Dermatoscopic magnifier**: Make sure it is in good working order and within easy reach.
- **Gloves**: Wear them during the examination, especially if you plan to touch sensitive lesions or areas.
- **Other instruments**: Have scissors, forceps or other tools available in case a biopsy or other sampling is required.

6. Patient positioning
- **Comfortable position**: Place the patient in a relaxed, comfortable position, depending on the area to be examined.
- **Access to areas to be examined**: Ensure that areas of interest are easily accessible and well lit.

7. Informed consent
  - If a procedure, such as a biopsy, is envisaged during the examination, it is crucial to obtain the patient's informed consent. This involves explaining the nature, risks, benefits and alternatives of the procedure, and ensuring that the patient understands and agrees.

Preparing the patient for a dermatological examination is an essential step in ensuring an accurate diagnosis and optimal treatment. It aims to put the patient in the best possible conditions, while ensuring their comfort and safety. Careful preparation contributes to the success of the examination and to patient satisfaction.

Biopsy assistance and other minor operations

Biopsies and other minor dermatological procedures are often necessary to establish a precise diagnosis or to treat certain skin lesions. The care assistant plays an essential role in these procedures, supporting the dermatologist and ensuring the patient's comfort and safety. Here is a detailed overview of this support role.

1. Before the operation
  - **Preparation of equipment**: Ensure that all the necessary instruments are ready and sterilised. This may include needles, scalpels, forceps, tubes for samples, etc.
  - **Preparing the area to be operated on**: Clean and disinfect the area of skin concerned. Apply an antiseptic, then place a sterile field around the area.
  - **Patient comfort**: Place the patient in a comfortable and reassuring position, briefly explain the procedure and ensure that they are relaxed.

2. During the operation
  - **Assisting the dermatologist**: Passing instruments requested by the dermatologist in a sterile manner, helping with lighting or adjusting the patient's position if necessary.
  - **Patient monitoring**: Carefully observe the patient's reaction, check for signs of discomfort or stress, and communicate any concerns to the dermatologist.
  - **Sample management**: If a biopsy is performed, ensure that the sample is correctly placed in a tube or container, labelled and ready to be sent to the laboratory.

3. After the operation
  - **Wound care**: Apply a sterile dressing to the area to be treated. Depending on the procedure, an antibiotic cream or other medication may be required.
  - **Post-procedure advice**: Inform the patient about the care to be given to the surgical area, the signs of infection to be monitored and the possible need for a follow-up visit.
  - **Cleaning**: Ensure that all instruments used are properly cleaned and sterilised for future use. Dispose of all medical waste correctly.

4. Pain and comfort management
  - **Local anaesthetic**: If a local anaesthetic is used, make sure that the patient is comfortable and feels no pain during the procedure.
  - **Post-procedure**: Ask about the patient's pain or discomfort. Depending on the dermatologist's instructions, analgesics may be recommended.

Assisting with a biopsy or other minor procedure is a crucial aspect of the dermatology orderly's role. By working closely with the dermatologist and ensuring that the patient is well cared for, the orderly contributes to the success of the procedure and the achievement of accurate diagnostic results.

Management and care of wounds and sutures

Care of wounds and sutures is essential to ensure optimal healing and prevent infection. In dermatology, many procedures, from biopsies to excisions, may require sutures. The nursing auxiliary has a vital role to play in the post-operative management of these wounds. Here is a detailed exploration of this responsibility.

1. Initial wound assessment
   - **Observation of the wound**: Examine the wound for signs of infection, such as excessive redness, swelling, purulent discharge or an unpleasant odour.
   - **Pain control**: Ask the patient about their pain level and inform the dermatologist if an intervention is necessary.

2. Cleaning the wound
   - **Gentle technique**: Use a saline solution to gently clean the wound, avoiding vigorous rubbing which could damage the newly formed tissue.
   - **Avoid alcohol and peroxide**: These substances can delay healing by damaging healthy cells.

3. Application of medicines
   - **Antiseptics**: Apply a mild antiseptic if recommended by the dermatologist.
   - **Creams or ointments**: Some may be prescribed to reduce the risk of infection or to promote healing.

4. Dressings
- **Choice of dressing**: Use the type of dressing recommended for the specific type of wound. For example, a moist wound may require a hydrocolloid dressing.
- **Regular change**: Replace the dressing as recommended by the dermatologist or as soon as it becomes soiled or wet.

5. Suture care
- **Cleaning**: Gently clean the area around the sutures with a saline solution or as instructed by the dermatologist.
- **Monitoring**: Observe sutures regularly for signs of pulling, loosening or infection.
- **Patient education**: Inform the patient not to pull or scratch the sutures and to report any discomfort or problems.

6. Follow-up and removal of sutures
- **Follow-up visits**: Organise follow-up appointments to check the healing of the wound and the condition of the sutures.
- **Removal**: Assist the dermatologist with suture removal, ensuring the wound is sufficiently healed.

7. Patient education and advice
- **General advice**: Instruct the patient on how to care for the wound at home, in particular by avoiding submersion in water, protecting the wound from the sun, and avoiding any tension or rubbing on the area.
- **Signs of infection**: Educate the patient about the signs of infection or complications, and tell them when to contact the clinic or doctor.

Careful management of wounds and sutures is crucial to the patient's recovery from dermatological procedures.

Thanks to their supportive role, nursing auxiliaries play a central role in this phase of care, ensuring the patient's well-being and optimal results.

Chapter 4:
INTERACTIONS WITH PATIENTS

The importance of empathic communication

Dermatology, like all medical fields, requires effective communication between the healthcare professional and the patient. However, given that skin conditions are often visible and can have a profound psychosocial impact on the patient, empathic communication is particularly crucial. Let's take a closer look at the importance of this essential skill in dermatology.

1. Definition of empathic communication
   - **Recognition**: The ability to recognise and understand the feelings and perspectives of others.
   - **Validation**: This involves validating and accepting the patient's emotions without judgement.
   - **Emotional response: This** involves responding in a way that demonstrates genuine understanding and appreciation of the patient's concerns.

2. Why is this crucial in dermatology?
   - **Psychological impact of skin conditions**: Skin problems can have a profound effect on a person's self-esteem, confidence and quality of life. Empathetic communication helps to mitigate these impacts.
   - **Trust**: Patients are more likely to trust a healthcare professional who demonstrates empathy, which facilitates the therapeutic relationship.

- **Compliance with treatment**: Patients who feel understood and supported are more likely to follow medical recommendations.

3. Empathetic communication techniques
   - **Active listening**: concentrating entirely on the patient when they are speaking, without interrupting or judging.
   - **Reflection**: Repeat or paraphrase what the patient says to show that they are being heard.
   - **Open questions**: Encourage patients to share their feelings and concerns by asking questions that require more than a simple "yes" or "no" answer.
   - **Non-verbal language**: Use appropriate eye contact, open posture and gestures to show interest and concern.

4. Benefits for healthcare professionals
   - **Better understanding**: By establishing empathic communication, the healthcare professional can obtain a more complete and nuanced picture of the patient's situation.
   - **Job satisfaction**: Creating genuine links with patients can increase job satisfaction and a sense of achievement.
   - **Preventing burnout**: Empathetic communication can help reduce stress and emotional fatigue by strengthening positive links with patients.

5. Challenges and considerations
   - **Training**: Although empathy is partly innate, empathic communication techniques can require training and practice.
   - **Emotional balance**: Too much empathy can be emotionally draining for the professional. Finding a balance between connecting with the patient and

maintaining a certain emotional distance is essential for the mental health of the carer.

Empathetic communication is a cornerstone of effective and caring dermatological care. By recognising and validating patients' emotional experiences, healthcare professionals can create strong therapeutic relationships and help patients successfully navigate their care pathways.

Understanding and managing the patient's pain and anxiety

Pain and anxiety are common experiences for many dermatology patients. Whether it is an invasive procedure or anxiety related to a skin condition, understanding and managing these emotions is essential to providing holistic care. In this chapter, we will explore the nature of pain and anxiety in dermatology and how healthcare professionals, particularly healthcare assistants, can respond empathetically and effectively.

1. The nature of pain and anxiety in dermatology
   - **Physical pain**: Can be caused by procedures such as biopsies, excisions or wound treatment.
   - **Emotional pain**: Distress linked to physical appearance or the social stigma associated with certain skin conditions.
   - **Anxiety**: Fear of procedures, worry about diagnosis, stress related to managing a chronic illness.

2. Recognising signs of pain and anxiety
   - **Verbal**: Complaints of pain, frequent questions, trembling voice.
   - **Non-verbal**: Muscle tension, grimaces, closed posture, avoidance of eye contact.

- **Behavioural**: Irritability, agitation, insomnia, mood swings.

3. Communication techniques for understanding pain and anxiety
  - **Active listening**: Lending an attentive ear to the patient's concerns without interruption.
  - **Open questions**: Encourage patients to express their feelings.
  - **Validation**: Recognising and validating the patient's emotions without judgement.

4. Management strategies
  - **Relaxation techniques**: deep breathing, guided visualisation, progressive muscle relaxation.
  - **Distraction**: Music, reading, light conversation to distract attention from pain or anxiety.
  - **Information**: Informing the patient about what to expect during the procedure or treatment can reduce anxiety.
  - **Medication**: If necessary, discuss with the dermatologist the possibility of using analgesics or anxiolytic drugs.

5. The role of the care assistant
  - **Emotional support**: Being a reassuring presence, offering a hand to hold, or simply being there to listen.
  - **Preparation and reassurance**: Explaining the stages of a procedure and reassuring the patient about the measures taken to minimise pain.
  - **Monitoring**: Observe signs of pain and anxiety and report them promptly to the dermatologist or medical team.

6. Importance of continuing training
  - **Updating skills**: Techniques and methods for managing pain and anxiety are evolving. Ongoing training enables care assistants to keep up to date.
  - **Emotional support for carers**: Managing patients' pain and anxiety can be emotionally demanding for carers themselves. Finding ways to recharge their batteries is crucial.

Understanding and managing pain and anxiety is essential to providing comprehensive dermatology care. By adopting a proactive and empathetic approach, healthcare professionals can help patients navigate these difficult experiences with dignity and confidence.

Educating the patient : prevention and home care

Patient education is a fundamental pillar of dermatological care. Not only does it help to improve patients' understanding of their disease or condition, it also helps them to adhere to treatment and prevent complications. For the dermatology carer, it is essential to know how to effectively educate the patient about prevention and home care.

1. The importance of patient education
  - **Autonomy**: Well-informed patients are better equipped to make informed decisions about their care.
  - **Adherence to treatment**: A clear understanding of the reasons for and benefits of treatment increases the likelihood of adherence.
  - **Preventing complications**: Informed patients are better able to recognise the early signs of complications and seek help.

2. Prevention in dermatology
   - **Sun protection**: Teaching the importance of regular use of sunscreen, the choice of appropriate protection and best practice in its application.
   - **Skin hygiene**: Discuss best practices for cleansing and moisturising the skin, as well as recommended products for different skin types.
   - **Skin self-examination**: Instruct patients on how and when to carry out a skin self-examination to detect early changes.

3. Home care for various skin conditions
   - **Eczema**: Advice on moisturisers, warm baths, reducing triggers.
   - **Psoriasis**: Information on topical treatments, the importance of hydration and avoiding triggers.
   - **Acne**: Education on appropriate facial care, products to avoid and regular treatment.
   - **Wounds and sutures**: Advice on cleaning, monitoring for signs of infection and general wound care.

4. Use of visual resources
   - **Brochures and leaflets**: Provide printed materials that patients can take home and consult.
   - **Videos**: Use educational videos to demonstrate care techniques or explain concepts.
   - **Models and mock-ups**: Sometimes, three-dimensional models of the skin or devices can help clarify the instructions.

5. Effective communication techniques
   - **Open questions**: Encourage the patient to ask questions to make sure they understand.
   - **Repetition**: Repeat key information to reinforce understanding.

- **Feedback**: Ask the patient to summarise or demonstrate what they have learned to confirm understanding.

6. The role of the care assistant
   - **Reinforcement**: Reiterate the key information shared by the dermatologist.
   - **Demonstration**: Showing the patient how to apply a medicine or perform a specific treatment.
   - **Assessment**: Make sure the patient has understood by asking for feedback or observing their actions.

Patient education is a shared responsibility between all members of the dermatology care team. The carer plays a vital role in ensuring that the patient has the knowledge and skills to manage their condition effectively at home. Effective education leads to better outcomes for the patient and greater satisfaction for the healthcare professional.

Chapter 5:
COLLABORATE
WITH THE MEDICAL TEAM

Synergy with the dermatologist: understanding expectations

Working in a dermatology department involves close collaboration between the dermatologist and the care assistant. This synergy is essential to ensure optimal patient care. For this collaboration to be successful, the healthcare assistant must understand and meet the dermatologist's expectations. This chapter will focus on the importance of this professional relationship and how it can be cultivated and maintained.

1. The unique role of the dermatologist
   - **Diagnosis and treatment**: Understanding the specific skills and responsibilities of the dermatologist in determining skin pathologies and their treatment.
   - **Consultation and follow-up**: Assessment of the importance of regular consultations and follow-up to monitor disease progression and treatment effectiveness.

2. Key expectations of the dermatologist
   - **Preparing the patient**: Ensure that the patient is properly prepared for the examination, both physically and emotionally.
   - **Technical assistance**: Helping with procedures, whether by passing instruments, illuminating the examination area or assisting with biopsies.

- **Effective communication**: Report any observations or feedback from the patient that may be relevant to the dermatologist.
- **Patient education**: Complementing the dermatologist's explanations of treatments or home care.

3. Open and regular communication

- **Daily discussions**: Take the time to discuss cases, concerns or observations with the dermatologist.
- **Team meetings**: Actively participate in meetings to stay informed and share relevant information.

4. Cultivating trust

- **Competence**: Continuing to train and develop skills to ensure optimum patient care.
- **Integrity**: Being honest about your observations, even if they differ from those of the dermatologist.
- **Reliability**: Being regular and punctual, showing predictability in your actions and the quality of your work.

5. Understanding the dermatologist's perspective

- **Pressures and responsibilities**: Recognising the issues that the dermatologist may face, such as difficult cases or time constraints.
- **Need for efficiency**: Helping the dermatologist to maximise his or her efficiency by anticipating needs.

6. The role of the care assistant in strengthening collaboration

- **Initiative**: Suggesting improvements or adjustments to procedures or care to improve efficiency or patient comfort.
- **Feedback**: Regular feedback from the dermatologist on performance and areas for improvement.

The collaboration between the healthcare assistant and the dermatologist is a delicate dance of skills, communication and trust. By clearly understanding the dermatologist's expectations and actively working to meet those needs, the carer can strengthen this vital professional relationship, resulting in better patient care and a more rewarding working experience for both parties.

Interaction with nurses and other medical staff

The complexity of the medical world requires seamless cooperation between all those involved. In a dermatology department, the nursing auxiliary frequently interacts with the nurses, but also with many other health professionals. This collaboration is crucial to ensuring that patients receive effective, holistic care.

1. The importance of multidisciplinary collaboration
   * **Exchange of expertise**: Each member of the team has a unique speciality and experience that can benefit the patient.
   * **Continuity of care**: Effective communication between professionals ensures that the patient receives consistent and continuous care.
   * **Optimising resources**: Working together means that available resources can be used more effectively and duplication avoided.

2. Interaction with nurses
   * **Complementary roles**: While nurses often administer medication and manage technical care, care assistants offer practical and emotional support.
   * **Information transfer**: Communication about the patient's condition, concerns or observed changes.

- **Care coordination**: Ensuring that treatment and care are administered in a timely and effective manner.

3. Working with physiotherapists
   - **Post-operative care**: In dermatology, certain treatments or procedures may require physiotherapy to promote healing or improve mobility.
   - **Practical advice**: Physiotherapists can provide recommendations on patient positioning or exercises to encourage.

4. Exchanges with pharmacists
   - **Drug clarification**: Understanding potential side effects, contraindications or drug interactions.
   - **Advice on administration**: Knowing how and when to administer treatments for maximum effectiveness.

5. Teamwork with laboratory technicians
   - **Specimen transfer**: Ensure safe and efficient transfer of biopsy specimens or cultures.
   - **Understanding results**: Interpreting test results to better inform patient care.

6. Communication with medical secretaries and administrative staff
   - **Appointment management**: Ensuring that patients receive reminders and updates about their upcoming consultations.
   - **Passing on information**: Communicating any changes in the patient's condition or care needs that may affect the timetable or resources.

7. Tips for effective collaboration
   - **Active listening**: Valuing the opinions and knowledge of other team members.
   - **Clear communication**: Use simple, precise language to avoid misunderstandings.

- **Mutual respect**: Recognising the value and expertise of each team member.

As an essential link in the care chain, the healthcare assistant plays a central role in promoting fruitful collaboration with other healthcare professionals. Effective communication and collaboration not only improve the efficiency of the service, but also ensure that the patient receives comprehensive and holistic care.

Transmission of information: medical records, reports, and verbal communications

The correct and efficient transmission of information is a cornerstone of the smooth running of a medical unit. In the dermatology department, the nursing auxiliary, like other health professionals, must be meticulous and attentive to this transmission to ensure optimum patient care.

1. Medical records: the basis for continuity of care
   - **File components**: Medical history, allergies, prescribed medication, past interventions, tests and results, consultation notes, etc.
   - **Updating the file**: The importance of adding recent and relevant information after each operation or consultation.
   - **Access and confidentiality**: Who can access the file, how it is protected, and why confidentiality is essential.

2. Writing and reading reports
   - **Types of reports**: Examination reports, post-operative reports, incident reports, etc.

- **Clarity and precision**: How to write reports that convey essential information without ambiguity.
- **The importance of proofreading**: Ensuring the accuracy and relevance of information before sharing it.

3. Verbal communication: the challenge of clarity
- **Handover meetings**: The importance of exchanging information between teams during changes of service.
- **Communicating with patients**: how to convey information in a way that is empathetic, reassuring and clear.
- **Interacting with other healthcare professionals**: Use professional, precise and respectful language.

4. Importance of digital documentation
- **Electronic medical record management systems**: how they work, their importance for consistency of care, and precautions to take when using them.
- **Secure data transmission**: Protocols to ensure that digital information is shared securely.

5. Managing situations where information is missing or ambiguous
- **Finding missing information**: Who to contact and how to check missing or ambiguous details.
- **Protocols for dealing with uncertainty**: How to proceed if you are uncertain about the relevance or accuracy of a piece of information.

6. Training and updating skills
- **The importance of ongoing training**: Keeping abreast of best practice in documentation and communication.

- **Resources and workshops**: Take advantage of internal and external training to improve your skills in transmitting information.

The effective transmission of information is essential to avoid medical errors, optimise patient care and ensure team cohesion. The nursing auxiliary, often at the interface between the patient and several medical professionals, plays a crucial role in this process. Appropriate training, constant attention and a commitment to precision and clarity are therefore essential.

Chapter 6:
CASE STUDIES IN DERMATOLOGY

Eczema:
understand, treat and assist

Eczema is one of the most common skin conditions encountered in dermatology. For a healthcare assistant working in this field, it is essential to understand this condition, to know the main treatments and to be able to provide appropriate support to affected patients.

1. What is eczema?
   - **Definition**: An inflammatory skin condition manifested by redness, itching and rashes.
   - **Types of eczema**: atopic eczema, contact eczema, seborrhoeic eczema, etc.
   - **Causes and triggers**: Allergies, irritants, genetic factors, stress, and other environmental elements.

2. Symptoms and diagnosis
   - **Common symptoms**: Red patches, intense itching, dry, scaly skin, oozing in some cases.
   - **Diagnostic process**: Anamnesis, clinical examination, allergy tests, and other investigations if necessary.

3. Common treatments
   - **Topical creams and ointments**: Steroids, immunomodulators, emollients.
   - **Antihistamines**: To reduce itching.
   - **Light therapy**: controlled exposure to specific types of light.

- **Skin hygiene advice**: Warm baths, use of gentle cleansers, regular moisturising.

4. The role of the nursing auxiliary in the management of eczema
  - **Assisting with treatments**: Helping to apply creams or lotions, assisting with light therapies.
  - **Patient education**: Providing information about eczema, treatments and best skin care practices.
  - **Emotional support**: Recognising and responding to the emotional distress associated with eczema, listening to patients' concerns.

5. Prevention and advice for everyday life
  - **Identifying and avoiding triggers**: Advice on products to use, clothes to wear and lifestyle habits to adopt.
  - **Regular moisturising**: Regular application of emollients is important to maintain the skin barrier.
  - **Stress management**: suggesting relaxation techniques, recommending resources or professionals if necessary.

6. Working with the medical team
  - **Updating medical records**: documenting the course of the disease, reactions to treatment and any other relevant observations.
  - **Communication with dermatologists**: sharing patients' concerns, finding out about treatment changes.

Eczema, although common, can have a significant impact on patients' quality of life. A well-trained and empathetic carer can play a crucial role in helping these patients to manage their condition, follow their treatments and find comfort in the challenges posed by this skin condition.

Psoriasis:
a comprehensive approach to care

Psoriasis is a chronic inflammatory skin disease which, although not contagious, can have a major impact on patients' quality of life. For a dermatology orderly, it is vital to understand this disease, the associated treatments and the need for holistic patient management.

1. Introduction to psoriasis
   - **Definition**: An immune disorder that accelerates the life cycle of skin cells.
   - **Types of psoriasis**: Plaque psoriasis, guttate psoriasis, erythrodermic psoriasis, pustular psoriasis and reverse psoriasis.
   - **Causes and triggers**: Genetics, immune system, environmental factors, infections, stress, etc.

2. Symptoms and diagnosis
   - **Common symptoms**: Red patches covered with silvery scales, dry, cracked skin, itching, pain.
   - **Diagnostic process**: Clinical examination, skin biopsy and sometimes blood tests.

3. Treatments for psoriasis
   - **Topical treatments**: Steroids, vitamin D, retinoids, etc.
   - **Systemic treatments**: Methotrexate, cyclosporine, acitretin, and others.
   - **Biotherapies**: Medicines that target specific parts of the immune system.
   - **Photodynamic therapy**: Use of UV light.

4. The role of the carer in the management of psoriasis
   - **Assistance with treatments**: Application of creams, preparation for phototherapy, etc.

- **Patient education**: Information on psoriasis, adherence to the treatment regime and skin care.
- **Emotional and psychological support**: Support in dealing with the stigma, anxiety and depression associated with the disease.

5. The global approach: beyond skin care
- **Managing co-morbidities**: Identifying and treating associated conditions, such as psoriatic arthritis.
- **Nutrition and lifestyle**: dietary advice, stress management, the importance of exercise.
- **Connectivity with support groups**: Encourage patients to join support groups or forums to share their experiences.

6. Working with the medical team
- **Updating medical records**: recording observations, the progress of the disease and any reactions to treatment.
- **Interdisciplinary communication**: Interacting with dermatologists, rheumatologists (for psoriatic arthritis) and other relevant specialists.

Managing psoriasis is not just about the skin. It requires a holistic understanding of the physical, emotional and social impact of the disease on patients. Caregivers play an essential role in this management, providing both clinical care and emotional support to help patients manage their condition in the best possible way.

Skin cancer:
roles and responsibilities care assistant

Skin cancers are among the most common types of cancer. Early detection and appropriate treatment are crucial to ensure the best chances of recovery. As part of the medical team, the nursing auxiliary plays a fundamental role, both in the day-to-day support provided to the patient and in assisting with medical interventions.

1. Understanding skin cancer
   - Types of skin cancer:
     - Basal cell carcinoma
     - Squamous cell carcinoma
     - Melanoma
     - Other rare forms
   - **Risk factors**: Sun exposure, family history, fair skin, age, certain pre-existing skin lesions, etc.

2. Symptoms and detection
   - **Warning signs**: Changes to a mole, appearance of new lesions, wounds that do not heal.
   - **Role of the care assistant**: Encourage regular self-examinations, identify and report any abnormalities.

3. Treatments and interventions
   - **Treatment options**: Surgery, radiotherapy, chemotherapy, immunotherapy.
     - The role of the care assistant during treatment:
     - Preparing the patient before an operation
     - Assistance during the procedure (if necessary)
     - Post-operative care and follow-up

4. Patient support
   - **Emotional management**: Helping the patient to cope with the fear, anxiety and uncertainty associated with the diagnosis.
   - **Physical support**: Helping with daily care, ensuring the patient's mobility and comfort.
   - **Education**: Providing information on preventive measures, post-treatment care and the necessary medical follow-up.

5. Prevention and awareness
   - **Sun protection**: Educate people about the importance of protection against UV rays.
   - **Early detection**: Raising awareness of the importance of regular skin checks.

6. Collaboration and communication with the medical team
   - **Passing on information**: Keeping the medical team informed about the patient's general condition, concerns and needs.
   - **Working in synergy**: Ensuring smooth communication with dermatologists, oncologists, nurses and other members of the healthcare team.

Skin cancers can be treated effectively if detected early. Caregivers, through their close contact with patients, play a crucial role in the detection, management and support of skin cancer patients. Properly trained and informed, they can make a major contribution to improving the patient's prognosis and quality of life.

Chapter 7:
DAILY CHALLENGES

Managing dermatological emergencies

Dermatological emergencies can manifest themselves in a variety of ways and require rapid intervention to avoid complications. For healthcare assistants working in dermatology, in-depth knowledge of these situations and how to manage them is essential. Their role is to support the medical team and ensure patient safety and comfort.

1. Recognising dermatological emergencies
   - **Acute eruptions**: Urticaria, erythema multiforme, drug reactions.
   - **Sudden skin infections**: cellulitis, abscess, necrotising fasciitis.
   - Rapid worsening of an existing disease: Severe eczema, erythrodermic psoriasis.

2. First steps
   - **Initial assessment**: Checking vital signs, assessing pain, identifying symptoms.
   - **Keeping the patient safe**: Ensuring a comfortable position, reassuring the patient, guaranteeing easy access to oxygen and emergency medicines if necessary.
   - **Rapid notification**: Inform the medical team of the situation immediately.

3. Assistance with emergency treatment
   - **Preparing medicines**: Rapid preparation of prescribed treatments (antihistamines, antibiotics, steroids, etc.).

- **Interventional support**: Assisting with biopsies, drainages and other interventions where necessary.

4. Post-intervention monitoring
- **Ongoing observation**: Monitor vital signs, evolution of the rash or lesion and response to treatment.
- **Communication with the patient**: Regularly checking on pain levels and comfort, and answering the patient's questions.

5. Education and prevention
- **Post-emergency advice**: Inform the patient about home care, signs of aggravation and the need for follow-up.
- **Preventing recurrences**: Educate about potential triggers, drugs to avoid and protective measures.

6. Documentation and transmission
- **Incident reports**: Document the event in detail, the interventions carried out and the patient's response.
- **Communication with the medical team**: Ensuring the smooth transmission of information to guarantee continuity of care.

When faced with a dermatological emergency, the speed of action and skill of the healthcare assistant can make a significant difference to the outcome for the patient. Working closely with the medical team, the nursing auxiliary provides vital support for the effective management of these critical situations.

Emotional charge: understanding and managing burn-out

The medical environment, with its high demands and often stressful situations, exposes healthcare professionals in particular to the risk of burn-out. For care assistants, who are often on the front line interacting with patients, the emotional burden can be particularly heavy. Understanding this phenomenon and putting in place prevention strategies is essential to ensure the well-being of these professionals.

1. Definition and recognition of burn-out
   - **What is burn-out? Burn-out is an** advanced form of burnout, characterised by diminished energy, disillusionment and reduced professional effectiveness.
   - Symptoms :
     - Emotional: irritability, anxiety, depression.
     - Physical: chronic fatigue, sleep disorders, headaches.
     - Behavioural: isolation, cynicism, reduced performance.

2. Contributing factors specific to dermatology
   - **Exposure to distressed patients**: Many dermatological conditions affect patients' self-esteem, making their reactions more emotionally charged.
   - **Work schedule**: Dermatology can involve long working days, especially in emergency departments.

3. Prevention strategies
   - **Balance workload and rest periods**: make sure you take regular breaks and don't overload your schedule.
   - **Training and supervision**: Stress and emotion management training, as well as supervision or discussion groups, can help prevent burn-out.

4. The importance of communication
   - **With colleagues**: share your feelings, discuss the difficulties you've encountered and support each other.

- **With management**: Report any situation where you feel unwell or any early signs of burn-out, so that you can adapt your working conditions.

5. Psychological support
  - **Consult a professional**: If you are at risk of burn-out, it is essential to consult a psychologist or psychiatrist.
  - **Talking groups and peer support**: talking to colleagues in a protected setting is a great way to share your feelings and get support.

6. Resuming work after a burn-out
  - **Recognition and acceptance**: Recognising burn-out and accepting the need to rest and seek help.
  - **Adapting your working pace**: Considering part-time work, reviewing your organisation, delegating certain tasks.
  - **Reconstruction**: therapeutic work, relaxation activities, strengthening the social support network.

The emotional burden inherent in the profession of care assistant calls for heightened vigilance to prevent burn-out. By adopting preventive strategies, strengthening communication and seeking support, it is possible to navigate through the emotional challenges of the profession while preserving mental health.

Respect for confidentiality and professional ethics

In the medical field, professional ethics and respect for confidentiality are essential pillars guaranteeing a relationship of trust between patients and healthcare professionals. Healthcare assistants, who are in direct and regular contact with patients, have a crucial responsibility in this respect.

1. Confidentiality: a fundamental right
   - **Definition and scope**: Confidentiality is the duty to keep personal or medical information about a patient secret, except in very specific cases.
   - **Why we exist** : Protecting privacy, respecting human dignity, and maintaining confidence in the healthcare system.

2. Confidentiality issues in dermatology
   - **Sensitive information**: Dermatological problems can affect a patient's intimacy, self-esteem and identity.
   - **Psychological implications**: A breach of confidentiality can have serious consequences for a patient's mental health, which is why it is so important to maintain confidentiality.

3. Principles of professional ethics
   - **Benevolence**: Always acting in the patient's best interests.
   - **Integrity**: Being honest and transparent in our actions and communications.
   - **Autonomy**: Respecting patients' decisions and treating them as active participants in their own care.
   - **Justice**: Ensuring equal treatment for all patients.

4. Day-to-day application
   - **Data protection**: Ensure that medical records are secure, do not discuss patients in public.
   - **Appropriate communication**: Only share information if necessary and only with the healthcare professionals concerned.
   - **Discreet conversations**: Avoid discussions about patients in communal areas or with colleagues not involved in the patient's care.

5. Common ethical dilemmas
  * **Conflict of interest**: Always put the patient's well-being first, even if this may conflict with personal or institutional interests.
  * **Patient requests vs. medical protocol**: How should you react when a patient requests a non-conventional treatment or approach?

6. Continuing education and ethical reflection
  * **Take part in training courses**: Ongoing training keeps you up to date with ethical issues and best practice.
  * **Focus groups**: Take part in focus groups or seminars on ethics to discuss complex cases or dilemmas.

Respecting confidentiality and professional ethics is a major responsibility for healthcare assistants. These principles, which are fundamental in the medical field, ensure that a relationship of trust is maintained between the patient and the care team, which is essential to the quality of the care provided.

Chapter 8:
DEVELOPMENT AND TRAINING

Opportunities
continuing education

Continuing education is an essential part of any healthcare professional's career. For dermatology nursing assistants, this means not only maintaining and broadening their skills, but also going into specific areas in greater depth, ensuring quality of care and responding to constant changes in the medical environment.

1. Why pursue continuing education?
   * **Developments in the medical field**: Medicine and dermatology are constantly evolving, with new techniques, new treatments and new discoveries.
   * **Regulatory requirements**: Some countries require a certain number of hours of continuing education to maintain certification or accreditation.
   * **Professional development**: broaden your skills, specialise or consider a career move.

2. Types of training available
   * **Clinical training**: on specific techniques, new treatments or recent technologies.
   * **Theoretical training**: on anatomy, pathophysiology or specialised areas of dermatology.
   * **Cross-disciplinary training**: stress management, communication, medical ethics, medical IT.

3. Training methods
   * **Traditional courses**: face-to-face, in training centres or academic institutions.

- **Online training**: webinars, MOOCs, instructional videos.
- **Practical workshops**: simulations, role-playing, work in small groups.
- **Conferences and seminars**: Presentations of recent research, exchanges with other professionals, workshops.

4. Recognising quality training
- **Accreditation**: Ensure that training is recognised by professional bodies.
- **Qualified trainers**: Favour training given by experts recognised in their field.
- **Feedback**: Consult the opinions of other participants.

5. Financing continuing education
- **Professional grants**: Many institutions offer scholarships or grants for continuing education.
- **Public funding**: Some states offer grants for the continuing education of healthcare professionals.
- **Self-financing**: Investing personally in your training is also a commitment to your career.

6. Possible career paths and specialisations
- **Specialisations**: Focusing on a specific area of dermatology (paediatric dermatology, skin oncology, etc.).
- **Career options**: Become a trainer, move into research, or consider positions of greater responsibility in the medical field.

Continuing education is a valuable opportunity for dermatology orderlies. It enables them to hone their skills, keep up to date with constant innovations and ensure that the care they provide is always of the highest possible quality.

Specialisation in dermatology

Dermatology, although a medical speciality in its own right, offers multiple sub-specialities and areas of expertise. For a healthcare assistant wishing to specialise further, it is essential to understand these various niches in order to guide their continuing education and career.

1. Why specialise?
   - **Depth of knowledge**: Acquire in-depth expertise in a specific area of dermatology.
   - **Responding to a specific request**: Certain dermatological disorders require special expertise.
   - **Career development**: Specialisation can open doors to positions of greater responsibility or areas of research.

2. The different sub-specialities in dermatology
   - **Paediatric dermatology**: Specialising in skin diseases of children and infants.
   - **Dermato-oncology**: focused on the diagnosis, treatment and prevention of skin cancers.
   - **Surgical dermatology**: Focuses on surgical procedures to treat various skin conditions.
   - **Cosmetic dermatology**: Focusing on aesthetic procedures and treatments to improve the appearance of the skin.
   - **Immunological dermatology**: Focuses on skin diseases linked to the immune system, such as lupus or psoriasis.

3. Training and certification
   - **Specialised courses**: Many institutions offer courses focusing on a particular sub-specialty.
   - **Certifications**: After training, obtaining certification in a sub-specialty can add value to a CV.

- **Work placements and internships**: Working directly in a sub-specialty offers invaluable practical experience.

4. Collaboration with specialist dermatologists
   - **Understanding specific needs**: Each sub-specialty has its own needs and requirements.
   - **Adapting to specific technologies and treatments**: Surgical dermatology, for example, may require familiarity with certain instruments or techniques.

5. Specialisation challenges and rewards
   - **Challenges** : The need for ongoing training, keeping abreast of the latest research and advances in the sub-specialty.
   - **Rewards**: Satisfaction of being an expert in a field, ability to provide highly specialised care, and potentially higher remuneration.

6. Professional considerations
   - **Job opportunities**: Some medical centres and hospitals may be looking for specialist care assistants.
   - **Networking**: Attend conferences or seminars related to your chosen sub-specialty to establish contacts in the field.

Specialising in dermatology for a healthcare assistant is a promising route for those looking to further their knowledge and provide highly specialised care. With the constant evolution of medicine and the diversity of skin conditions, there are a multitude of opportunities for those willing to invest in their training and career.

The professional network: importance and development

A solid, well-maintained professional network is an invaluable tool in the medical field and, in particular, for a dermatology orderly. Not only does it give you access to new opportunities, it also allows you to share best practice, get advice and receive support when you need it.

1. Why is it important to build up a professional network?
   - **Professional exchanges**: Discussing medical advances, new techniques and challenges encountered.
   - **Career opportunities**: Access to job offers, recommendations and promotions.
   - **Training and development**: Find out about relevant training courses, workshops or upcoming seminars.
   - **Emotional support and mentoring**: Benefit from advice, feedback and support in the event of doubts or difficulties.

2. How do you build your professional network?
   - **Initial training:** Training colleagues, trainers and lecturers.
   - **Workplace**: Colleagues, doctors, nurses, administrative staff.
   - **Professional associations**: Membership of nursing auxiliary or dermatology groups.
   - **Conferences and seminars**: Meetings with experts in the field, exchanges with colleagues from other institutions.
   - **Professional social networks**: Platforms like LinkedIn allow you to connect with professionals from all walks of life.

3. How do you maintain your network?
- **Regular contacts**: Send occasional messages, share articles or relevant information.
- **Taking part in events**: Attend conferences, workshops, seminars or meetings.
- **Offer help**: Offer support or expertise whenever possible. Helping each other strengthens professional ties.
- **Professional updates**: Inform your network of changes in your career, new certifications or acquired skills.

4. Mistakes to avoid
- **Neglecting your network**: An unmaintained network can weaken over time.
- **Only ask when you need to**: A relationship should be a two-way street. You shouldn't just call on your network when you need help.
- **Not being grateful**: Always thank and show gratitude to those who offer help or advice.

5. The impact of a solid network on a career
- **Career development**: A good network can open doors to unexpected opportunities.
- **Broadening skills**: Through exchanges with experts or colleagues from other institutions, you can learn and integrate new skills or techniques.
- **Confidence and self-assurance**: Knowing that you have a solid network behind you can boost your confidence in your abilities and decision-making.

Building and maintaining a professional network is a long-term investment in your career. For a dermatology orderly, this means having access to a wealth of information, support and opportunities that can greatly benefit their career path.

Chapter 9:
TESTIMONIES AND LIFE STORIES

A typical day in the life of a care assistant in dermatology

Dermatology, with its variety of pathologies and treatments, presents a busy and varied day for a healthcare assistant. Here's an overview of a typical day for a care assistant working in the dermatology department of a hospital or clinic.

6.30 - 7.00: Arrival and preparation
- **Check-in**: Registration of arrival at the hospital or clinic.
- **Preparation**: Dressing (gown, gloves, mask if necessary).
- **Briefing with the team**: overview of the day's appointments, planned operations and hospitalised patients.

7.00am - 9.00am: Morning care
- **Visiting in-patients**: checking vitals, administering prescribed care, checking dressings.
- **Preparation of examination rooms**: Ensure that all the necessary equipment is ready and sterilised.

9.00am - 12.00pm: Consultations
- **Welcoming patients**: Settling into the examination room, taking vital signs, checking medical records.
- **Assistance with examinations**: Presence during the consultation to help the dermatologist (lighting, equipment, etc.).

- **Post-consultation care**: Application of creams or dressings, explanations to the patient about home care.

12:00 - 13:00: Lunch break

1.00 pm - 4.00 pm: Minor operations
- **Preparing the patient**: Cleaning and disinfecting the area to be treated.
- **Assistance during the operation**: Passing instruments, helping to keep the patient in the right position.
- **Post-op care**: Application of dressings, advice on post-operative care.

16.00 - 18.00: End-of-day care
- **Visiting patients in hospital**: checking dressings, administering medication.
- **Cleaning and disinfection**: Ensuring that examination rooms are clean and ready for the next day.

6.00 pm - 6.30 pm: Transmission
- **Briefing with the evening team**: Passing on important information about hospitalised patients and any incidents that may have occurred during the day.
- **Updating medical records**: Ensuring that all records are up to date with the day's procedures and treatments.

6.30pm: End of the day

Of course, this routine may vary depending on the size of the facility, the number of patients and the procedures planned. A dermatology department in a large hospital will undoubtedly have a different dynamic to a small private clinic. However, whatever the structure, the ability to adapt and manage several tasks simultaneously is essential for a dermatology orderly.

Highlights:
challenges and successes

Being a dermatology orderly involves daily interaction with patients from a wide range of backgrounds, and every day can bring its share of challenges and successes. Here are a few examples of the highlights of a dermatology orderly's career.

1. Challenges
   - **Severe cases of acne in teenagers** : Acne, although common, can have profound emotional implications, especially in teenagers. Assisting a dermatologist in treating severe cases and seeing a young patient in distress can be difficult. The challenge lies in providing emotional support to the patient while ensuring effective medical care.
   - **Diagnosis of skin cancers**: Taking part in the diagnosis and management of patients with skin cancers such as melanoma can be an intense experience. Compassion and support are essential to help these patients through this ordeal.
   - **Managing dermatological emergencies**: When faced with severe allergic reactions, acute skin infections or other emergencies, speed and efficiency are essential. These situations can test the skills and composure of the nursing auxiliary.

2. Success stories
   - **Long-term follow-up**: Seeing a patient improve over months or even years is one of the greatest rewards of the job. This can be the case for chronic conditions

such as psoriasis or eczema, where the patient returns regularly for treatment.

- **Patient education**: Educating patients about skin care, the dangers of sun exposure and the importance of regular screening, and seeing them incorporate this advice into their daily lives is a major achievement.
- **Participating in successful procedures**: Assisting the dermatologist during procedures, whether excisions, biopsies or other treatments, and seeing the positive result on the patient is a proud moment.
- **Emotional support**: Sometimes success lies not only in medical care but also in the human aspect. Offering emotional support to an anxious patient, reassuring a frightened child or simply listening to someone's concerns can have a profound impact on their well-being.

Being a dermatology carer, while demanding, offers many opportunities to celebrate successes and learn from challenges. These milestones shape careers, build resilience and serve as a constant reminder of the importance of the carer's role in the patient's care pathway.

Lessons learned
past experience

In the medical world, and particularly as a dermatology orderly, every day is a learning opportunity. Experiences, both positive and negative, provide valuable lessons for the future. Here are some key lessons that can be learned from past experiences:

1. The importance of listening :
Sometimes patients need to talk, to express their fears or concerns. Learning to really listen, without judging or

interrupting, is essential. Not only does this lead to better care, it also helps to establish a relationship of trust with the patient.

2. The need for continuing education :
Dermatology, like other medical fields, is evolving rapidly. New treatments, techniques and emerging research make continuing education essential. Each past experience underlines the importance of staying up to date in your field.

3. The value of patience :
Not all patients respond in the same way to treatment. Some may show rapid improvements, while others require more time. Patience is therefore an essential virtue.

4. The importance of teamwork :
Nobody works alone in the medical world. Past experience shows how crucial it is to communicate well with colleagues, whether they are other orderlies, dermatologists, nurses or administrative staff.

5. The human aspect above all :
Medicine is not just a science, it's also an art. Human interaction is at the heart of this profession, and every patient is unique. Past experience reminds us that beyond symptoms and diagnoses, there is a person with his or her emotions and needs.

6. The need for self-care:
In the face of stress, emotional strain and long hours, the importance of self-care becomes obvious. In order to help others, you first have to look after your own well-being.

7. The importance of thoroughness and organisation :
Details count, especially in healthcare. Whether it's

preparing a patient, updating a medical file or keeping a room clean, thoroughness is essential.

8. Learn from your mistakes:
Nobody is perfect. Everyone makes mistakes, but the important thing is to recognise them, learn from them and try not to repeat them.

These lessons, drawn from past experience, form the basis of a rewarding and successful career in dermatology. They serve as a reminder that, although science and technique are at the heart of this profession, the human aspect remains paramount.

Chapter 10:
TOOLS AND TECHNOLOGIES
IN DERMATOLOGY

Presentation
commonly used equipment

Dermatology, as a medical speciality, requires a variety of specialist equipment to examine, diagnose and treat skin conditions. Dermatology orderlies need to be familiar with these tools to effectively assist the dermatologist and care for the patient. Here is an overview of the equipment commonly used in this field:

1. The dermatoscope :
This device allows the skin to be examined on an enlarged scale. It is often used to assess moles and other skin lesions to detect early signs of melanoma or other skin cancers.

2. Wood's light lamp :
This is a special lamp that emits ultraviolet light. It is used to diagnose skin conditions such as fungal infections, pigmentation disorders and other conditions that may appear differently under this type of light.

3. Electrosurgical equipment :
These use electric current to cut or destroy tissue. They can be used to remove warts, moles or other small skin lesions.

4. Cryosurgical devices:
These devices use extreme cold (usually liquid nitrogen) to freeze and destroy skin lesions, such as warts.

5. Light therapy equipment :
Some skin disorders, such as psoriasis, can be treated with special lights. Dermatology practices may have special rooms or cabinets for light therapy.

6. Biopsy equipment:
This includes scalpels, punches and other tools needed to take a small sample of skin which will then be examined in the laboratory.

7. Laser equipment:
Many dermatological treatments, such as tattoo removal, scar reduction or vascular therapy, use specialist lasers.

8. The examination table with adjustable light:
Essential for any dermatology practice, this table allows the dermatologist to examine the patient from different angles and light intensities.

9. Dressing materials:
Includes bandages, compresses, antiseptics and other supplies needed to clean, treat and cover wounds or incisions.

10. Other disinfection equipment :
Autoclaves and other sterilisation equipment ensure that all tools and equipment are properly disinfected before each use.

Familiarity with this equipment is essential for dermatology orderlies. Not only does it help to ensure the safety and effectiveness of care, but it also reinforces the patient's confidence in the quality of the care they receive.

The role of the nursing auxiliary in maintenance and sterilisation

The maintenance and sterilisation of medical equipment are crucial to ensuring the safety of patients and medical staff. In dermatology, where procedures can often be invasive, this importance is accentuated. The nursing auxiliary plays an essential role in these processes.

1. Preparing instruments for sterilisation :
   - **Sorting**: After use, the nursing auxiliary sorts the instruments according to their type and material.
   - **Preliminary cleaning**: Instruments are first cleaned to remove coarse matter, such as blood or other secretions.

2. Use of the autoclave :

The autoclave is the most commonly used device for sterilising medical instruments. The care assistant must :
   - Load the autoclave correctly.
   - Select the right cycle for the type of instrument.
   - Ensure that the autoclave reaches the correct temperature and pressure.
   - Regularly check that the appliance is working properly.

3. Checking sterilisation :

After sterilisation, the orderly must:
   - Inspect the instruments to make sure they are clean.
   - Check the autoclave sterilisation indicator or use biological tests to confirm sterilisation.

4. Storage of sterilised instruments :

Instruments must be stored in a clean, dry place, protected from contamination. The care assistant must ensure that they are correctly packaged and labelled with the sterilisation date.

5. Regular maintenance of equipment :
The care assistant is often responsible for :
- Daily checking of equipment.
- Report any malfunctions.
- Carry out routine maintenance, such as changing filters or checking seals.

6. Compliance with protocols and regulations :
Each medical establishment has specific protocols for sterilisation and maintenance. Healthcare assistants must be trained in these protocols and ensure that they are strictly adhered to.

7. Ongoing training :
Sterilisation methods and technologies are evolving. Healthcare assistants need regular training to keep up to date with best practice.

8. Personal protection :
The safety of the caregiver is equally important. This means wearing appropriate personal protective equipment, including gloves, masks and goggles when handling dirty instruments or during the sterilisation process.

The nursing auxiliary's role in maintenance and sterilisation is vital to ensuring the safety and efficiency of dermatology care. The responsibility that this entails demands competence, rigour and a constant commitment to the quality of care.

Technological innovations and their impact on day-to-day work

Technological developments have always played a decisive role in the medical field. In dermatology, these innovations are transforming not only the treatments available, but also the way care assistants and other professionals interact with patients and with each other.

1. Improved diagnostics :
   - **Advanced imaging**: Imaging technologies such as digital dermoscopy and magnetic resonance imaging (MRI) offer detailed views of skin conditions.
   - **Skin analysis applications**: These applications allow patients to scan areas of their skin using smartphones and send the images for preliminary analysis.

2. Customised treatments :
   - **Gene therapy and biotechnology**: These technologies enable targeted treatments for conditions such as psoriasis or eczema based on the patient's genetics.
   - **New-generation lasers**: More precise and less invasive, these lasers reduce recovery times and minimise scarring.

3. Telemedicine :
   - **Virtual consultations**: Patients can now consult dermatologists remotely, which means that care assistants have to adapt to this method of communication and help to set up the necessary equipment.
   - **Remote monitoring**: Some devices allow you to monitor the progress of a skin condition from a distance.

4. Augmented and virtual reality :
   - **Training and simulation**: These technologies offer healthcare assistants more immersive and realistic training opportunities.
   - **Diagnostic aid**: Augmented reality can help visualise skin conditions by superimposing them on the patient's own skin.

5. Automation and robotics :
- **Automated equipment**: Some equipment can now be programmed to perform repetitive tasks, such as instrument preparation and sterilisation.
- **Robotic assistance**: In some cases, robots assist doctors during operations, requiring specific training for nursing assistants.

6. Advanced information systems :
- **Electronic medical records**: Digitising medical records makes them easier to access and update.
- **Monitoring applications and platforms**: These tools enable patients and professionals to track the progress of a condition or treatment in real time.

7. Impact on daily work :
- **Ongoing training**: Healthcare assistants need regular training to understand and use these new technologies effectively.
- **Adapting to new procedures**: Daily routines can be altered by the introduction of new technologies, requiring adaptability.
- **Improved patient interaction**: Thanks to technology, care assistants can provide more personalised care and respond more quickly to patients' needs.
- **Increased efficiency**: Innovations can often simplify or speed up certain tasks, allowing care assistants to concentrate on other aspects of care.

Technological innovations will continue to evolve and impact the field of dermatology. Nurses, like all healthcare professionals, must embrace these changes while ensuring that the quality and humanity of care is maintained.

Chapter 11:
PAEDIATRIC DERMATOLOGY

Special   features and challenges working with children

Working with children, particularly in a medical context such as dermatology, presents unique characteristics and challenges. Children are not simply "little adults"; their understanding, reactions and needs are different from those of adults.

1. Cognitive understanding :
   - **Developmental level**: Children of different ages have different levels of comprehension. It is crucial to present information in a way that is adapted to their cognitive level.
   - **Fear of the unknown**: Children can be frightened by environments or procedures they don't understand. It is essential to reassure them.

2. Communication :
   - **Appropriate language**: Caregivers must use clear, simple language, often accompanied by examples or analogies suitable for children.
   - **Visuals**: Illustrations, toys or books can help explain a procedure or illness.

3. Emotional reactions :
   - **Variability**: Children can move quickly from one emotional state to another. Crying, anxiety or anger may come on suddenly.

- **Need for reassurance**: Nurses often have to adopt a reassuring, even maternal role, to calm and reassure the child.

4. Cooperation :
    - **Distractions**: Using toys, videos or music can help distract a child during an examination or procedure.
    - **Parental involvement**: Parents or guardians can play an essential role in reassuring the child and facilitating cooperation.

5. Physiological considerations :
    - **Skin reactions** : Children's skin may react differently to treatments or tests than that of adults.
    - **Dosage**: Dosages of medicines or creams should be adjusted according to the child's weight and age.

6. Infrastructure and equipment :
    - **Appropriate size**: Whether it's chairs, beds or instruments, everything must be adapted to the size and comfort of the children.
    - **Warm environment**: A brightly coloured environment, with toys or drawings, can make the space more welcoming for children.

7. Liaison with other specialists :
    - **Child psychology**: Care assistants may need to work with mental health specialists to help traumatised or extremely anxious children.

8. Training and preparation :
    - **Specialist training**: Working with children may require specific paediatric training or certification.
    - **Role-playing**: Simulations or role-playing can prepare care assistants for the unique challenges of caring for children.

Working with children in dermatology requires patience, adaptability and empathy. Each child is unique, and the approach must be individualised to ensure effective and caring care. Healthcare assistants must constantly evolve and learn to meet the specific needs of this population.

Common skin conditions in children

Children's skin is often faced with specific challenges linked to their age, environment and development. Many skin conditions are common in childhood. Here's an overview of the most common:

1. Atopic dermatitis (eczema) :
   * **Description: This is a** chronic inflammation of the skin that causes itching and redness.
   * **Causes**: Although it can be linked to genetics, atopic dermatitis is often aggravated by environmental triggers such as dryness, cold or certain allergens.

2. Varicella :
   * **Description**: Viral disease characterised by a pruritic, vesicular rash.
   * **Causes**: Caused by the varicella-zoster virus.

3. Impetigo :
   * **Description**: Superficial bacterial infection of the skin producing red patches often covered with yellowish crusts.
   * **Causes**: Mainly caused by the bacteria Staphylococcus aureus or Streptococcus pyogenes.

4. Warts :
   * **Description**: Rough, non-cancerous growths that generally appear on the hands and feet.

- **Causes**: Caused by the human papillomavirus (HPV).

5. Ringworm (tinea) :
   - **Description**: Fungal infection that can affect different parts of the body, such as the scalp or feet, causing round, scaly patches.
   - **Causes**: Caused by dermatophytes, a type of fungus.

6. Angiomas (haemangiomas) :
   - **Description**: Birthmarks or small masses that appear shortly after birth, often red or purplish.
   - **Causes**: Caused by the proliferation of blood vessels in a specific area of the skin.

7. Milium :
   - **Description**: Small white or yellowish cysts that often appear on the face of infants.
   - **Causes**: Result from obstruction of the sweat glands on the surface of the skin.

8. Prickly heat (diaper rash) :
   - **Description**: Reddish skin rash, often seen in areas covered by babies' nappies.
   - **Causes**: It is generally due to irritation caused by moisture, friction or contact with urine and faeces.

9. Roseole :
   - **Description**: Viral disease characterised by high fever followed by a pink rash.
   - **Causes**: Usually caused by the human herpesvirus 6 (HHV-6).

10. Molluscum contagiosum :
    - **Description**: Small, often dome-shaped, growths on the skin which may be pale, whitish or pinkish.
    - **Causes**: Caused by the molluscum contagiosum virus.

It is essential to diagnose and treat these conditions correctly. Parents need to be educated about the causes, symptoms and treatments available, as well as preventative measures to avoid the spread or recurrence of these conditions. Collaboration between carers, dermatologists and parents is crucial to ensuring children's skin health.

Communication
and collaboration with parents

When it comes to treating skin conditions in children, collaboration with parents or guardians is crucial. They are usually the ones who will observe the first symptoms, administer treatments and provide the necessary follow-up. Here are some key points concerning communication and collaboration with parents in paediatric dermatology:

1. Building trust :
   * **First contact**: First impressions are important. Parents' concerns must be actively listened to, and they must be reassured of their essential role in the care process.
   * **Empathy**: Recognising and validating parents' emotions. Their sick child can be a source of considerable anxiety.

2. Open communication :
   * **Clear language**: Avoid complex medical jargon. Provide information in a simple, understandable way.
   * **Questions**: Encourage parents to ask questions and be sure to answer fully and patiently.

3. Education :
- **Explanations**: Explain in detail the nature of the skin condition, the possible causes, the symptoms to look out for and the treatment steps.
- **Documentation**: Provide brochures, fact sheets or online references to help parents better understand and follow the advice at home.

4. Involvement in decision-making :
- **Treatment options** : Present the different options available, their advantages and disadvantages.
- **Feedback**: Encourage parents to share their observations and concerns about their child's treatment or reaction.

5. Ongoing collaboration :
- **Regular follow-up**: Schedule follow-up appointments to assess the progress of the condition and the effectiveness of the treatment.
- **Accessibility**: Make sure parents know how to contact you if they have any questions or concerns between appointments.

6. Respect for privacy :
- **Confidentiality**: Ensure that medical information is treated with the utmost respect for the family's confidentiality and privacy.
- **Informed consent**: Make sure parents understand the procedures, tests or treatments before giving their consent.

7. Emotional support :
- **Reassurance**: Parents may feel guilty or responsible for their child's skin condition. It's important to reassure them and provide emotional support.

- **Support network**: Refer parents to support groups or resources that can help them manage their stress and worries.

8. Promoting prevention :
   - **Home advice**: Provide advice on hygiene routines, products to use or avoid, and steps to take to avoid triggers.
   - **Raising awareness**: Inform parents about the early signs of skin disorders so that they can intervene quickly.

The success of paediatric dermatology treatment depends to a large extent on effective communication and close collaboration with parents. A patient- and family-centred approach will ensure optimal care for the child.

Chapter 12:
GERIATRIC DERMATOLOGY

Ageing skin:
special features and needs

The skin ageing process is inevitable and is influenced by many factors, both intrinsic and extrinsic. Understanding the changes that occur with age and the specific needs of ageing skin is essential for appropriate dermatological management.

1. Physiological changes :
   - **Thinner skin**: With age, skin becomes thinner due to a reduction in collagen production.
   - **Loss of elasticity**: The reduction in elastic fibres leads to a loss of elasticity, resulting in sagging skin and the formation of wrinkles.
   - **Increased dryness**: The skin's ability to retain moisture decreases, leading to increased dryness and can cause itching.

2. Vascular changes :
   - **Capillary fragility**: The skin becomes more prone to bruising and subcutaneous haemorrhaging.
   - **Reduced circulation**: Reduced circulation can lead to delayed healing and increased susceptibility to ulcers.

3. Pigment alterations :
   - **Age spots (solar lentigos)**: These pigmented spots generally appear on areas exposed to the sun, such as the face, hands and arms.

- **Dark circles**: These can darken with age due to the increased thinness of the skin and vascular changes.

4. Tumours and growths :
   - **Seborrhoeic keratoses:** benign, rough, brownish growths.
   - **Actinic keratoses:** Pre-cancerous lesions caused by excessive exposure to the sun.
   - **Skin tumours**: Older people are more likely to develop skin cancers such as basal cell carcinoma, squamous cell carcinoma and melanoma.

5. Specific needs :
   - **Moisturising**: Rich moisturising products are essential for maintaining the integrity of the skin barrier.
   - **Sun protection**: Ageing skin needs ongoing protection against the harmful effects of UV rays.
   - **Nutrition**: A balanced diet rich in antioxidants can help maintain skin health.
   - **Specialist treatments**: Depending on needs, treatments may include fillers, botulinum toxins, laser therapy and cosmetic surgery.

6. Drug sensitisation :
   - Many medicines can have side effects on the skin. It is therefore important to monitor the skin of elderly people undergoing medication.

7. Education and prevention :
   - Raising awareness among the elderly of the importance of regular skin self-examinations to detect changes.
   - Encourage regular dermatological visits for early detection of skin disorders.

Caring for ageing skin requires an in-depth understanding of the physiological changes and associated challenges. A proactive, preventive approach, combined with appropriate skin care, will help to maintain the health and integrity of the skin throughout the ageing process.

Common skin conditions in the elderly

With age comes a host of changes in the skin, making it more vulnerable to a variety of conditions. Here is a list of common skin conditions in older people, with a brief description of each:

1. Xerosis (dry skin) :
   - This is one of the most common skin complaints among the elderly. It is characterised by rough, scaly or cracked skin, often due to a reduction in the skin's ability to retain moisture.

2. Pruritus (itching) :
   - Often associated with xerosis, pruritus can also be caused by other skin conditions, medication or systemic diseases.

3. Actinic keratoses :
   - These rough, scaly lesions are potential precursors of squamous cell carcinoma and result from cumulative exposure to the sun.

4. Seborrheic keratoses :
   - These are benign, flesh-coloured to brown lesions with a warty surface. They can appear anywhere on the body.

5. Dermatoporosis :
  * The skin is extremely fragile, often showing signs of easy bruising and pseudocicatricial lesions.

6. Senile purpura :
  * These are bruises that appear easily, especially on the forearms and backs of the hands, due to the fragility of the blood vessels.

7. Malignant skin tumours :
  * These include basal cell carcinoma, squamous cell carcinoma and melanoma. Sun exposure, family history and advanced age are risk factors.

8. Varicose veins :
  * These dilated and twisted veins, often visible on the legs, are the result of wear and tear on the valves of the veins.

9. Pressure ulcers :
  * These ulcers are caused by prolonged pressure on a specific area of the skin, usually where the bones are close to the skin, such as the heels or elbows.

10. Herpes zoster (shingles) :
  * Shingles is a painful skin rash caused by reactivation of the varicella-zoster virus. Older people, particularly those with weakened immune systems, are more likely to develop shingles.

11. Fungal infections :
  * Yeast and other fungal infections are common, especially in warm, moist areas of the body such as the feet or skin folds.

12. Abrasion :
  * Superficial wounds caused by repeated rubbing, such as as wearing ill-fitting shoes.

13. Age spots (solar lentigos) :
   * These pigmented spots, which are generally harmless, are caused by prolonged exposure to the sun.

14. Acanthosis nigricans :
   * Thickened, pigmented areas, often in skin folds, may be associated with metabolic disorders such as diabetes.

It is crucial for the elderly and their carers to recognise these conditions, understand their nature and consult a dermatologist if necessary. Regular monitoring and adequate protection can help prevent or effectively treat many common skin conditions in the elderly.

Holistic approach: collaborate with other medical specialities

Dermatology, although focused on the skin, is not isolated from the rest of the body. The skin is a reflection of general health, and many skin conditions can be a sign of systemic problems. For this reason, a holistic approach to dermatology means working closely with other medical specialities to provide comprehensive care for the patient.

1. Introduction: The importance of an integrated approach
   * The interconnection between the skin and the body's other systems.
   * Recognition of skin disorders as potential symptoms of systemic diseases.

2. The relationship with endocrinology
  - Skin conditions linked to hormonal imbalances, such as acne, pigmentation disorders during pregnancy or acanthosis nigricans linked to diabetes.
  - Importance of working together to adjust hormone treatments.

3. Collaboration with rheumatology
  - Autoimmune diseases such as lupus or scleroderma can have cutaneous manifestations.
  - Skin biopsy as a diagnostic tool for rheumatic diseases.

4. Working with gastroenterologists
  - Liver or intestinal diseases, such as hepatitis or coeliac disease, can manifest themselves as rashes or itching.
  - Importance of liver function tests in certain dermatological treatments.

5. Synergy with cardiology
  - Some dermatological medicines can have an effect on the cardiovascular system.
  - Cyanosis, a cutaneous sign of hypoxia, requiring cardiac assessment.

6. Link with nephrology
  - Kidney disease can cause itching or urate deposits in the skin.
  - The implications of certain dermatological drugs on renal function.

7. Interaction with psychiatry
  - Management of conditions such as psoriasis or vitiligo that can affect mental health.
  - Dermatillomania, a compulsive skin disorder requiring a psychiatric approach.

8. Collaboration with oncologists
   * Joint management of patients with skin cancers, in particular melanomas.
   * Implications of chemotherapy on the skin and hair.

9. Conclusion: Towards interdisciplinary medicine
   * The importance of continuing training for dermatologists in systemic pathologies.
   * The benefits of regular communication between specialties for optimum patient care.

Dermatology is much more than just a skin speciality; it requires a holistic view of the patient. Interdisciplinary collaboration can not only lead to faster diagnosis, but also to more comprehensive care and better results for the patient.

Chapter 13:
PREVENTION AND EDUCATION IN DERMATOLOGY

The importance of prevention in skin health

As the largest organ in the human body, the skin plays a vital role in providing a protective barrier against external aggression, while regulating temperature and sensation. Skin health prevention is crucial not only for maintaining healthy skin, but also for preventing potentially serious illnesses.

1. Introduction :
   - The skin's role in protecting the body.
   - Consequences of damaged or diseased skin.

2. UV protection :
   - Risks associated with excessive exposure to the sun: premature ageing, skin cancer, cataracts.
   - The importance of wearing sunscreen, protective clothing and hats.
   - Awareness of maximum sunlight hours.

3. Daily skin care :
   - Gentle cleaning without over-washing or using aggressive products.
   - Regular moisturising to prevent dryness and cracks.
   - Recognising the signs of allergy or irritation caused by cosmetic products.

4. Diet and skin health :
  * Impact of a balanced diet rich in antioxidants, vitamins and minerals.
  * Link between dehydration and skin health.
  * Influence of certain foods and drinks on skin conditions such as acne or rosacea.

5. Stress management :
  * Influence of stress on the skin: rashes, itching, premature ageing.
  * Stress reduction techniques: meditation, yoga, exercise.

6. Importance of regular dermatological examinations :
  * Early detection of skin anomalies or cancers.
  * It's important to check your skin for any suspicious changes.

7. Protection in specific environments :
  * Skin care in extreme climates: heat, cold, humidity.
  * Precautions for workers exposed to chemicals or irritants.

8. Prevention of skin infections :
  * The importance of disinfecting cuts and scratches.
  * Recognition and early treatment of infections such as impetigo or athlete's foot.

9. Education and awareness :
  * The importance of educating children from an early age about skin care.
  * Raising public awareness of the risks of certain practices, such as sunbeds.

10. Conclusion :
  * Prevention is the key to healthy, resilient skin.

- Healthy daily choices can prevent a variety of skin problems, promote general well-being and boost self-confidence.

Skin health prevention is not just about a simple skincare routine, but encompasses a range of practices integrated into our daily lifestyle. Well-maintained skin is not only aesthetically pleasing, it also reflects optimal overall health.

The role of the nursing auxiliary in patient education

Patient education is a fundamental component of healthcare, enabling individuals to understand their condition, actively participate in their own care and improve their quality of life. As front-line healthcare professionals, healthcare assistants play an essential role in this educational process.

1. Introduction :
   - The importance of patient education in the care pathway.
   - The nursing auxiliary's unique position as a trusted communicator.

2. Assessment of the patient's educational needs :
   - Determining the patient's current level of understanding.
   - Identification of barriers to learning: language, culture, cognitive deficits.

3. Transmission of basic information :
   - Explanation of daily care routines.
   - Advice on nutrition, hygiene and exercise adapted to the patient's condition.
   - Clarification of myths and misconceptions.

4. Teaching home care techniques :
- Demonstration and practice of wound care techniques.
- Instructions for administering medication or applying topical treatments.
- Advice on preventing complications.

5. The importance of clear communication :
- Use of simple, understandable language.
- Use of visual tools or practical demonstrations.
- Regular checks on the patient's understanding.

6. Skin sensitisation :
- Education on the dangers of excessive exposure to the sun.
- Advice on choosing the right skincare products.
- Importance of self-examination to detect any abnormalities.

7. Education on warning signs :
- Recognising signs of infection, allergy or other complications.
- Instructions on when and how to contact a healthcare professional in an emergency.

8. Emotional and psychological support :
- Active listening to the patient's concerns and worries.
- Provide resources for psychological support, if necessary.

9. Working with the medical team :
- Sharing information about the patient's educational needs with other healthcare professionals.
- Regular updating of information to ensure consistent, up-to-date education.

10. Continuing education for care assistants :
   * Caregivers need to keep abreast of the latest advances and recommendations.
   * Participation in training courses and workshops to improve patient education skills.

11. Conclusion :
   * The vital role of the carer in empowering patients through education.
   * Positive impact of education on care outcomes and patient satisfaction.

Patient education is a complex task that requires patience, understanding and effective communication. Care assistants, thanks to their daily proximity to patients, are ideally placed to pass on crucial information, support patients in their care and thus contribute to better health outcomes.

Raising awareness of the dangers of the sun and other risk factors

Exposure to the sun is one of the biggest concerns in dermatology. Although the sun is essential for the production of vitamin D and promotes well-being, overexposure can lead to serious risks for the skin. At the same time, other environmental risk factors can also compromise skin health. It is therefore vital to raise public awareness of these dangers.

1. Introduction :
   * The importance of sunlight for health.
   * Harmful effects of excessive exposure.

2. Ultraviolet (UV) rays and their effects :
   * The difference between UVA and UVB rays.

- Impact of UV rays on the acceleration of skin ageing.
- Increased risk of skin cancer, including melanoma.

3. Sunburn and immediate dangers :
   - Symptoms and consequences of sunburn.
   - Risk of permanent damage and long-term complications.

4. The importance of sun protection :
   - Regular use of broad-spectrum sunscreens with an appropriate SPF.
   - Wear protective clothing: hats, sunglasses, long-sleeved clothing.
   - Seeking shade during the hottest hours.

5. Tanning beds and their risks :
   - Dangers of exposure to artificial UV rays.
   - Significant increase in the risk of skin cancer.
   - Banned and regulated in many countries.

6. Other environmental risk factors :
   - Pollution and its effects on the skin.
   - Exposure to chemicals or irritants.
   - The effects of smoking on skin health.

7. Skin recognition and self-examination :
   - The importance of regular skin monitoring.
   - Recognising the warning signs of skin cancer.
   - Consultation in the event of a change in a mole or the appearance of a new lesion.

8. Targeted awareness-raising :
   - Protecting children and raising awareness from an early age.
   - Specific precautions for people with fair skin, a family history or numerous moles.

9. Awareness campaigns and initiatives :
   * Advertising campaigns and educational programmes.
   * Free or reduced rate screening days.
   * Partnerships with organisations, schools and businesses to raise awareness among a wider audience.

10. Conclusion :
   * Prevention is the best defence against the dangers of the sun and other risk factors.
   * It is important to combine daily protection with regular monitoring to ensure optimum skin health.

Raising awareness of these dangers is not only essential for preventing skin conditions, but also for fostering a culture of preventive care, where everyone is aware of the risks and takes proactive steps to protect their skin.

Chapter 14:
MANAGING DIFFICULT SITUATIONS

Non-cooperative patients
or aggressive: how do you manage?

The world of healthcare is full of challenges, not least the management of difficult patients. It is crucial for medical staff, including healthcare assistants, to be equipped to manage uncooperative or aggressive patients to ensure their own safety, that of the patient and that of the team.

1. Introduction :
   * Recognising the stress and emotions that can lead to non-cooperation or aggression.
   * The importance of safety in the medical context.

2. Identify the cause :
   * Differentiating between non-cooperative and aggressive behaviour.
   * Identify possible sources of discomfort, pain or misunderstanding.
   * Understanding of possible medical reasons, such as neurological disorders, medication side-effects or delirium.

3. Preventive approach :
   * Creating a calm and welcoming environment.
   * Communicate clearly and regularly with the patient.
   * Establish a relationship of trust.

4. De-escalation techniques :
   * Active listening.
   * Validation of the patient's emotions without justifying the behaviour.

- Use a calm, reassuring tone of voice.
- Maintain a non-threatening posture.
- Avoid direct confrontation.

5. Physical interventions :
- Use as a last resort and only if safety is at stake.
- Knowledge and training in non-harmful restraint techniques.
- Ensuring the patient's well-being, even during a physical operation.

6. Call in the team :
- Ask for help as soon as you need it.
- Use the emergency bell system or the alert protocol.
- Clear communication with the team about the patient's behaviour.

7. After the incident :
- Assessment of the situation with the team.
- Discussions and debriefing to understand what happened and how to avoid similar incidents in the future.
- Take into account the emotional impact on staff and offer support where necessary.

8. Documentation :
- Keep accurate records of incidents, interventions and follow-up.
- Use of notes to inform the team, reassess care and as a basis for discussions with family or guardians.

9. Training and preparation :
- The importance of ongoing training for staff.
- Participation in training courses on managing aggression and conflict.
- Case studies and simulations to reinforce skills.

10. Conclusion :
* Recognition that non-cooperation or aggression is not usually directed at staff, but is often the result of fear, pain or confusion.
* The importance of empathy, patience and training to ensure the safety and well-being of all.

Managing a difficult patient is a challenge, but with the right skills, training and support, healthcare assistants can ensure the safety and well-being of patients while maintaining their own mental and emotional health.

Working with patients with skin conditions severe or disfiguring

Dermatology goes far beyond simple skin imperfections. Some patients suffer from severe, even disfiguring conditions, which can have a major impact on their self-esteem, quality of life and social interactions. For a carer, working with these patients requires a caring, sensitive and professional approach.

1. Introduction :
* Understanding the seriousness and psychosocial impact of severe or disfiguring skin conditions.
* The importance of empathy and respect in care.

2. Recognising the emotional impact :
* Psychological implications: shame, isolation, depression.
* Understanding the feeling of "loss of identity" or "bereavement" that some patients may experience.

3. Empathic communication approach :
* The importance of active listening.

- Avoid minimising or trivialising their concerns.
- Use of neutral, non-stigmatising terms.

4. Appropriate physical care :
   - Specialised techniques and products for severe conditions.
   - Gentle and delicate care to avoid pain or discomfort.
   - Being informed about current treatments and the patient's specific needs.

5. Creating a comfortable environment :
   - Ensuring confidentiality and discretion during care.
   - Use screens, curtains or private areas for treatment and examinations.

6. Psychological support :
   - Working closely with psychologists or counsellors.
   - Identify signs of emotional distress and recommend appropriate help.
   - Encourage participation in support groups or online communities.

7. Educate on the condition :
   - Helping patients to understand their condition.
   - Provide resources and information on treatment options and prospects.
   - Reassurance about medical advances and ongoing research.

8. Encouraging independence and self-care :
   - Teaching patients how to look after their skin at home.
   - Encourage self-care routines to improve self-confidence.

9. The importance of the interdisciplinary team :
   - Working with dermatologists, surgeons, psychologists, etc.

- Ensuring that all the patient's needs, both physical and psychological, are taken care of.

10. Taking care of yourself as a carer :
  - Recognising the emotions and stress associated with working with patients with serious medical conditions.
  - Seek support, take breaks and practise self-care.
  - Participate in training courses and discussion groups to share experiences and strategies.

11. Conclusion :
  - Working with patients with severe or disfiguring skin conditions is both demanding and rewarding.
  - By taking a holistic approach, carers can transform the lives of these patients, helping them to navigate both the physical and emotional challenges of their condition.

Caring for these patients requires a combination of medical expertise, communication skills and genuine humanity. Providing them with integral support can not only help treat their skin condition, but also restore their confidence and quality of life.

Emotional support :
for the patient and for yourself

In the world of healthcare, the clinical and medical aspects of care can sometimes overshadow the importance of emotional support. However, in the field of dermatology, where conditions can have a visible and therefore psychological impact, this support is vital. To provide this support effectively, care assistants not only need to be trained to understand and respond to patients' emotional needs, but also to take care of their own emotions.

1. Understanding the patient's emotional needs :
   - **Identifying signs of distress**: Learning to recognise the signs of emotional distress in a patient.
   - **Impact of skin conditions**: Understanding how certain skin conditions can affect self-esteem, confidence and quality of life.

2. Empathic communication techniques :
   - **Active listening**: The power of simply listening without judgement.
   - **Reformulation and validation**: Showing the patient that their feelings are valid and understood.

3. Providing psychological support :
   - **Referrals**: Knowing when and how to refer a patient to a mental health specialist.
   - **Support groups**: Encourage patients to join groups where they can share their experiences and support each other.

4. Taking care of your own emotions as a carer :
   - **Recognising compassion fatigue**: Understanding the signs and symptoms of burn-out and emotional fatigue.
   - **Self-care strategies**: relaxation techniques, meditation, exercises and more to maintain emotional balance.

5. Working with other professionals :
   - **Teamwork**: Working with psychologists, social workers and other professionals to provide holistic support to patients.
   - **Training and seminars**: Attend training courses on emotional support to keep up to date with best practice.

6. Handling difficult situations :
  - **Patients in crisis**: how to intervene when the patient is in severe distress.
  - **Death or end-of-life situations**: providing support in the most trying situations, and knowing how to manage your own emotions.

7. Conclusion :
  - The importance of balancing emotional support for the patient and taking care of one's own emotions.
  - The recognition that taking care of yourself is essential to providing the best possible care for your patients.

Emotional support is at the heart of patient-centred care. Caregivers play a crucial role in ensuring that patients' emotional needs are taken into account, while preserving their own well-being to ensure quality care.

Chapter 15:
DERMATOLOGY
IN A MULTICULTURAL CONTEXT

Patient care
from diverse cultural backgrounds

In a globalised world, cultural diversity is omnipresent, including in healthcare environments. For a dermatology orderly, being aware of and respectful of cultural differences is essential to providing quality care and establishing a relationship of trust with the patient. The aim of this chapter is to raise awareness and equip healthcare assistants to provide care that is tailored to each individual.

1. Introduction :
   * **Cultural diversity**: understanding what it means and why it is important in the medical environment.

2. The importance of cultural sensitivity :
   * **Impact on diagnosis**: Understanding how cultural beliefs or practices can influence symptoms and the use of healthcare.
   * **Influence on treatment**: Respecting cultural preferences and beliefs can affect adherence to treatment.

3. Communication with the patient :
   * **Language barriers**: Techniques for communicating effectively when the patient does not speak the same language.
   * **Non-verbal signs**: Recognising and understanding the importance of gestures and facial expressions in different cultures.

4. Religious and spiritual considerations :
- **Care practices**: Certain rituals or beliefs can influence the way a patient wishes to be cared for.
- **Purification rituals**: How certain rituals can influence skin care or dermatological procedures.

5. Skin health in different cultures :
- **Common skin conditions**: Certain skin conditions may be more common or perceived differently in different cultures.
- **Cultural aesthetic practices**: tattoos, scarification and other body modifications and their influence on the skin.

6. Working with medical interpreters :
- **Roles and responsibilities**: When and how to use an interpreter.
- **Ensuring confidentiality**: Protecting sensitive patient information while working with an interpreter.

7. Appropriate education and prevention :
- **Adapting resources**: Ensuring that educational materials are understandable to patients from all backgrounds.
- **Understanding and respecting traditional remedies**: Some patients may use traditional treatments alongside Western medicine.

8. Continuous training :
- **Available resources and training**: Keeping abreast of best practice in managing patients from culturally diverse backgrounds.
- **Feedback**: Learning from past experience to improve future care.

9. Conclusion :
* The importance of individualised care that respects and values each patient's culture.

Respect for cultural diversity is not just a matter of ethics, but also a key element in providing quality care and building trust. By understanding and respecting each patient's beliefs and practices, the dermatology caregiver builds trust and promotes positive health outcomes.

Sensitivity and respect for cultural differences in skin care

Skin is a reflection of individual identity and history, shaped not only by biology but also by culture. The way in which different cultures perceive and care for the skin can vary considerably. In a medical environment, particularly in dermatology, it is crucial to adopt a culturally sensitive and respectful approach. This chapter is dedicated to educating healthcare assistants on the importance of these cultural differences and guiding them on how to deal with them.

1. Introduction :
* **Skin and identity**: Exploring the role of skin as a reflection of individual and cultural identity.

2. Diversity of beauty standards :
* **Skin tone**: Cultural preferences regarding skin colour and clarity.
* **Texture and characteristics**: Expectations and standards vary according to region and culture.
* **Cultural body modifications**: tattoos, scarification and other practices.

3. Traditional skin care :
  - **Natural and home remedies**: Ingredients and methods used in various traditions.
  - **Spiritual and ritual practices**: the role of skin in religious and cultural rites.

4. Cultural influences on skin disorders :
  - **Perception of certain conditions**: how conditions such as vitiligo or alopecia can be perceived differently in different cultures.
  - **Treatment and management**: Treatment choices can be influenced by cultural beliefs.

5. Respectful communication :
  - **Listening without judgement**: The importance of listening to patients' concerns with empathy.
  - **Avoiding stereotypes** : Recognise and set aside personal prejudices.

6. Adapted education :
  - **Use of culturally relevant examples**: Provide information using examples that resonate with the patient.
  - **Working with community leaders**: Working with respected figures to disseminate information about skin health.

7. Challenges and solutions :
  - **Language barriers**: using interpreters and taking cultural nuances into account.
  - **Negotiating between traditional and modern medicine**: finding a balance between Western dermatological care and traditional remedies.

8. Continuing education and professional development :
  - **Workshops and seminars**: The importance of ongoing training to stay informed and competent.

- **Cultural exchanges**: The opportunity to learn first-hand about other cultures through exchange programmes.

9. Conclusion :
  - To highlight the importance of cultural sensitivity in building trust, improving the quality of care and promoting better health outcomes.

Cultural sensitivity in skin care is an essential skill for all healthcare professionals. By adopting a respectful and informed approach, healthcare assistants can provide superior care while building trust with their patients.

Specific features of the skin linked to genetics and ethnicity

Skin is a direct reflection of our genetic and ethnic heritage. It can vary considerably in terms of colour, texture, sensitivity and response to different environmental factors. This chapter aims to educate healthcare assistants about the skin characteristics associated with genetics and ethnicity, in order to better understand and respond to the specific needs of patients.

1. Introduction :
  - **The skin, mirror of our heritage**: Understanding how genetics influence the structure and function of the skin.

2. Skin structure and function according to ethnic group :
  - **Melanocytes and pigmentation**: The importance of melanocytes in skin colour and their distribution according to ethnic groups.
  - **Skin barrier**: Variations in barrier thickness and function according to ethnicity.

3. Skin characteristics by ethnic group :
- **Caucasian skin:** Sun sensitivity, ageing, vascular particularities.
- **Asian skin**: Resistance to wrinkles, sensitivity to pigmentation spots, post-inflammatory reactions.
- **African and Afro-Caribbean skin**: Predisposition to certain conditions such as keloid, natural protection against the sun, but risks associated with voluntary depigmentation.
- **Latino and Hispanic skin**: Varied pigmentation, risk of melasma, post-inflammatory reactions.
- **Skin of the Middle East and Indian subcontinent**: Variability in pigmentation, predisposition to melasma, susceptibility to scarring.

4. Common skin conditions by ethnicity :
- **Pigmented skin diseases**: melasma, vitiligo, post-inflammatory hyperpigmentation.
- **Healing reactions**: Keloids, hypertrophic scars.
- **Follicular disorders**: Pseudofolliculitis barbae, pilonidal cysts.

5. Specific care and treatment :
- **Appropriate sun protection**: Understanding needs according to skin pigmentation.
- **Pigmentation treatments**: Selection of safe lightening products, peels, lasers.
- **Management of specific conditions**: Recommendations adapted to each ethnic group.

6. Dermatological challenges for non-Caucasian skin :
- **Limitations of clinical studies**: The lack of data on darker skin in dermatological research.
- **Cultural sensitivity**: The importance of understanding cultural practices and beliefs related to skin care.

7. Continuing training and awareness :
   * **Updating knowledge**: The importance of ongoing training to understand ethnic peculiarities.
   * **Inter-professional collaboration**: exchanging ideas with skin care experts from different ethnic groups.

8. Conclusion :
   * The importance of recognising and respecting genetic and ethnic differences in order to provide appropriate, individualised care.

Recognition of skin differences linked to genetics and ethnicity is essential to providing appropriate care. By being informed and adopting a respectful approach, healthcare assistants can ensure effective, personalised dermatological care for each patient.

Chapter 16:
THE IMPORTANCE
CONTINUITY OF CARE

Long-term patient monitoring: why it's crucial

Long-term follow-up of dermatology patients is essential for a number of reasons. It allows the effectiveness of treatments to be assessed, the progression of skin conditions to be monitored, complications or side effects to be detected early, and ongoing support to be provided to the patient. In this chapter, we will explore in detail why long-term follow-up is crucial in dermatology and how the carer plays a key role in this process.

1. Introduction :
   - **The continuum of care**: Understanding the concept of long-term follow-up as an integral part of medical care.

2. Assessment of treatment efficacy :
   - **Initial response to treatment**: Observe and record the first signs of improvement or stabilisation.
   - **Treatment adjustments**: The need to modify doses, change medication or adopt new therapeutic approaches depending on the patient's responses.

3. Monitoring chronic conditions :
   - **Progressive skin conditions**: monitoring diseases such as psoriasis, eczema or lupus to anticipate and manage flare-ups.
   - **Preventing complications**: Detecting signs of complications early so that you can intervene quickly.

4. Early detection of skin cancers :
   - **Regular monitoring**: Importance of regular check-ups for patients at risk or with a history of skin cancer.
   - **Early intervention**: The benefits of early treatment to improve prognosis.

5. Monitoring side effects and complications :
   - **Drug monitoring** : Identifying potential side effects of dermatological medications.
   - **Rapid intervention**: Taking action to manage or prevent major complications.

6. Psychological and emotional support :
   - **Skin diseases and self-esteem**: Understanding the impact of skin diseases on patients' psychological well-being.
   - **Role of the carer**: Offering support, listening, and advice to help patients manage emotional challenges.

7. Continuing patient education :
   - **Up-to-date information**: Keeping patients informed about the latest advances, new treatment options and best practice in skin care.
   - **Self-management and prevention**: Encouraging patients to play an active role in managing their skin health.

8. Conclusion :
   - **The central role of follow-up**: Reaffirming the importance of long-term follow-up as a central element of dermatology care, with an emphasis on collaboration between the patient, the carer and the dermatologist.

In dermatology, as in many medical fields, long-term follow-up is essential to ensure the best possible results for patients. The nursing auxiliary, often the first point of contact, plays a crucial role in guaranteeing this effective and appropriate follow-up.

Appointment management, reminders and follow-up

Managing appointments, reminders and follow-ups is crucial in the medical field, particularly in dermatology, where many patients require long-term follow-up. The healthcare assistant is often at the heart of this process, ensuring that patients receive the care they need in a timely manner. This chapter details the role and responsibilities of the carer in managing these administrative and organisational aspects.

1. Introduction :
   - **Continuity of care**: The importance of regular follow-up in dermatology.
   - **Coordination with other specialists**: The need to collaborate with other medical specialities when treating complex dermatological pathologies.

2. Scheduling and organising appointments :
   - **The first contact**: How the care assistant gathers initial information to set up an appointment.
   - **Schedule management**: Ensuring that the available slots correspond to the needs of the patient and the dermatologist.

3. Reminders to patients :
   - **Importance of reminders**: Why reminders are crucial for follow-up.
   - **Call-back methods**: Telephone calls, text messages, emails and other digital tools.
   - **Managing cancellations and postponements**: how to react and reschedule if necessary.

4. Pre-appointment preparation :
- **Updating medical records**: Ensure that all recent information is available for the appointment.
- **Preparing the equipment**: Organising the instruments or equipment needed for the appointment.

5. Post-appointment follow-up :
- **Report writing**: Document observations, recommendations and prescribed treatments.
- **Scheduling future appointments**: Ensuring that patients receive an appointment for their next follow-up or for any additional examinations.

6. Coordination with other healthcare professionals :
- **Referrals and consultations**: How and when to refer a patient to another specialist.
- **Sharing information**: Communication with other professionals to ensure comprehensive care.

7. Emergency and contingency management :
- **Prioritising cases**: Identifying and acting quickly in the event of a dermatological emergency.
- **Calendar management**: how to reorganise appointments to accommodate emergencies.

8. Conclusion :
- **The importance of rigour and organisation**: Reiterating the central role of the care assistant in coordinating and monitoring dermatology care.

The efficient management of appointments, reminders and follow-ups is fundamental to ensuring continuity of care in dermatology. By coordinating these aspects, the nursing auxiliary not only makes life easier for the patient, but also helps to improve organisation and efficiency within the dermatology department.

Working with other specialities
to provide comprehensive care
of the patient

Although dermatology is a speciality in its own right, it does not work in isolation. Often, skin conditions may be a symptom or consequence of other medical conditions or require multidisciplinary management. For the dermatology carer, understanding and collaborating with other medical specialties is essential to ensure holistic patient care.

1. Introduction :
   - **The interdisciplinary nature of medicine**: how dermatology fits into the vast network of medical care.
   - **The importance of collaboration**: how joint management can benefit the patient.

2. Links between dermatology and other specialities :
   - **Rheumatology**: Autoimmune diseases and their cutaneous manifestations.
   - **Endocrinology**: Skin problems linked to hormonal imbalances.
   - **Oncology**: Collaboration in the management of skin cancers.
   - **Allergology**: skin allergies and allergy tests.
   - **Plastic surgery**: repairs after skin surgery, skin grafts.
   - **Gastroenterology**: Link between intestinal diseases and skin conditions such as psoriasis.
   - **Paediatrics**: Skin diseases specific to childhood.

3. Interdisciplinary communication :
   - **Exchanging medical records**: the importance of updating and sharing information.
   - **Multidisciplinary meetings**: collaborative discussions on complex cases.

- **Management protocols**: Establish guidelines for joint management.

4. The role of the nursing auxiliary in collaboration :
   - **Appointment coordination**: Helping patients navigate interdisciplinary appointments.
   - **Communication**: acting as a bridge between the patient, the dermatologist and other specialists.
   - **Education**: Helping patients to understand the need for and role of each specialist in their care.

5. Challenges and solutions :
   - **Communication problems**: how to overcome communication barriers between specialities.
   - **Specialist availability**: Waiting time management and care coordination.
   - **Differences of opinion**: how to manage different medical viewpoints for the benefit of the patient.

6. Conclusion :
   - **Patient-centred care**: The importance of seeing the patient as a whole and not just through the prism of dermatology.
   - **The evolution of multidisciplinary care**: the benefits of collaboration for the future of medicine.

The medical world is a complex ecosystem in which every speciality has a role to play. For the dermatology orderly, understanding this network and working in close collaboration with other specialities is essential to guarantee complete and effective patient care.

Chapter 17:
CONCLUSION AND OUTLOOK

The impact and growing importance of the dermatology orderly

Introduction :
- **Current context**: The rapid development of the medical sector and the increase in demand for dermatology.
- **The central role of the nursing auxiliary**: How this professional has become an indispensable pillar in the dermatology department.

1. History of the dermatology nursing assistant profession :
- **Origins**: The emergence of the profession and its initial development.
- **Early responsibilities**: The main roles entrusted to the orderly when he or she first starts working in dermatology.

2. Broadening the scope of action :
- **Patient care**: Increasing involvement in patient reception, comfort and preparation.
- **Working closely with dermatologists**: Assisting with minor procedures, managing medical records and coordinating care.
- **Education and prevention**: The role of educating patients about prevention and post-intervention care.

3. Impact on quality of care :
- **Optimising dermatologists' time**: The nursing auxiliary takes on tasks that allow dermatologists to concentrate on diagnosis and treatment.

- **Improving the patient experience**: The nursing auxiliary provides a reassuring and constant presence for the patient, from reception to discharge.
- **Continuity of care**: The nursing auxiliary plays an essential role in post-intervention follow-up, ensuring that patients follow recommendations and receive adequate care.

4. Training and specialisation :
- **The need for ongoing training**: In view of the rapid developments in dermatology, care assistants must constantly update their skills.
- **Opportunities for specialisation**: The diversity of skin conditions and treatments offers areas of specialisation for the most enthusiastic care assistants.

5. Challenges and opportunities :
- **Professional recognition**: Despite their crucial role, care assistants can sometimes be underestimated. How can we raise the profile of this profession?
- **Technological development**: Innovations in dermatology may require adjustments to the role of the care assistant, offering both challenges and opportunities.

Conclusion:
- **A booming profession**: With the development of dermatology and the growing awareness of the importance of skin care, the role of the care assistant is more crucial than ever.
- **The future of the profession**: Reflections on the future potential and continuing impact of the care assistant in the world of dermatology.

At the heart of the dermatology department, the healthcare assistant is much more than a simple auxiliary. Their presence, skills and dedication have a direct impact on the quality of care, the efficiency of the department and the patient experience. Recognising and valuing this role is essential for the future of dermatology.

The dermatology of tomorrow: innovations and developments

Introduction :
- **The evolving landscape of dermatology**: How the convergence of technology, research and clinical practice is shaping the future of dermatology.

1. Technological advances :
- **Digital dermatoscopy**: The use of imaging technology for early and accurate detection of skin lesions.
- **Artificial intelligence and diagnosis**: How AI can help dermatologists identify and diagnose skin conditions.
- **Laser-assisted treatments** : New laser applications for the treatment of various skin conditions.

2. Innovative therapies :
- **Gene therapy**: How specifically targeting genes can offer solutions for genetic skin conditions.
- **Immunotherapy for skin cancers**: Using the patient's own immune system to fight the cancer.
- **Skin microbiome**: Understanding and exploiting the beneficial bacteria on the skin to treat various conditions.

3. Personalised approach to dermatology :
- **Molecular dermatology**: Treatment based on individual genetics.

- **Adaptive skincare products**: Creams and lotions designed specifically for the unique needs of each individual.
- **Applications and wearables**: Tracking devices for skin health, offering personalised recommendations.

4. Dermatology and the environment :
- **Effects of climate change**: How environmental changes are influencing skin disorders.
- **Environmentally-friendly products**: The move towards sustainable treatments and care products.

5. Training and education for the future :
- **Virtual reality training**: Using VR to train dermatologists in procedures and diagnostics.
- **The importance of continuing education**: Ensuring that professionals keep up to date with rapid advances in the specialty.

6. Multidisciplinary collaboration :
- **Dermatology and mental health**: Understanding the profound link between skin health and mental health.
- **Collaboration with other specialities**: How other medical fields can enrich and be enriched by dermatology.

Conclusion:
- **Preparing for the future**: As dermatology continues to evolve, healthcare professionals, from nurses' aides to dermatologists, need to adapt and prepare for an exciting and transformative future.

Dermatology, like all branches of medicine, is constantly evolving. Faced with global challenges and technological innovations, it is reinventing itself, offering new ways of treating and understanding the skin. Embracing these changes will improve the quality of care and quality of life for patients.

Closing remarks : dedication to skin care

The skin, the envelope that protects us, is the mirror of our soul, our health and the reflection of our emotions. It is our first line of defence against external aggression, but it is also the silent witness to our internal battles, be they physiological, psychological or emotional. Dermatology, much more than a medical science, is the art of understanding this complex web that stretches across every centimetre of our bodies.

Every dermatology orderly has a mission every day: to listen, observe, touch, understand and care. Their role, often underestimated, is fundamental. They are the first face that many patients see, the first ear that listens to their concerns, and the first hands that bring relief.

The message to take away from this book is the importance and nobility of the job of dermatology orderly. Throughout all the techniques, skills, emotions and challenges presented, there is one constant: dedication. An unwavering dedication to improving each patient's quality of life, relieving their pain, bringing clarity to their worries, and restoring their self-confidence.

This dedication is at the service of the skin, but also at the service of humanity. Because caring for the skin means caring for the whole person. Every intervention, every treatment, every moment of communication is a stone added to the edifice of confidence, hope and healing.

To all current and future healthcare assistants, this final word is a tribute to your passion, your commitment and your invaluable contribution to the world of healthcare. May you continue to light the way for those who, through their skins, seek comfort, understanding and well-being. May you always find the strength, support and resources you need to continue along this noble path.

May this book be a source of inspiration, knowledge and motivation for all those who choose to devote themselves to the service of skin and, by extension, to the service of humanity.